T0091581

COMMUNITY-BASED MENTAL HEALTHCARE FOR PSYCHOSIS

This eye-opening book explores the need for, and how to successfully organise, community mental health teams that provide in-home care and treatment for people experiencing mental health difficulties, particularly those suffering from psychosis.

With an emphasis on community-based care and democratic psychiatry, the book presents two paradigm shifts necessary to bring mental healthcare directly into the community. The first is shifting perceptions from thinking of patients to recognising those in need of care as members of the public, moving away from a biomedical diagnostic approach. The second shift is the provision of support for the community environment, its families, friends and neighbours to pave the way for hospitableness towards people with mental health issues in a way that encourages compassion, empathy and a respect for differences. Through clinical case material, anthropological and phenomenological methods and personal experience in community-based care, Peter Dierinck presents new models for sheltered housing and innovative ways for struggling individuals to secure paid work within a community system.

Community-Based Mental Healthcare for Psychosis is important reading for psychiatric professionals, clinicians, social workers, caregivers and all mental health professionals looking after psychiatric patients with complex care needs.

Peter Dierinck has worked since 1987 within psychiatric institutions in Belgium, for the most part in Psychiatrisch centrum Gent-Sleidinge on a ward for homeless people. Since 2018 he has also worked for vzw Psyche on a Flemish project 'Quartermaking', a method for inclusion in the community.

THE INTERNATIONAL SOCIETY FOR PSYCHOLOGICAL AND SOCIAL APPROACHES TO PSYCHOSIS BOOK SERIES
Series editor: Anna Lavis

Established over 50 years ago, the International Society for Psychological and Social Approaches to Psychosis (ISPS) has members in more than 20 countries. Central to its ethos is that the perspectives of people with lived experience of psychosis, their families and friends, are key to forging more inclusive understandings of, and therapeutic approaches to, psychosis.

Over its history ISPS has pioneered a growing global recognition of the emotional, socio-cultural, environmental, and structural contexts that underpin the development of psychosis. It has recognised this as an embodied psycho-social experience that must be understood in relation to a person's life history and circumstances. Evidencing a need for interventions in which listening and talking are key ingredients, this understanding has distinct therapeutic possibilities. To this end, ISPS embraces a wide spectrum of approaches, from psychodynamic, systemic, cognitive, and arts therapies, to need-adapted and dialogical approaches, family and group therapies and residential therapeutic communities.

A further ambition of ISPS is to draw together diverse viewpoints on psychosis, fostering discussion and debate across the biomedical and social sciences, as well as humanities. This goal underpins international and national conferences and the journal *Psychosis,* as well as being key to this book series.

The ISPS book series seeks to capture cutting edge developments in scholarship on psychosis, providing a forum in which authors with different lived and professional experiences can share their work. It showcases a variety of empirical focuses as well as experiential and disciplinary perspectives. The books thereby combine intellectual rigour with accessibility for readers across the ISPS community. We aim for the series to be a resource for mental health professionals, academics, policy makers, and for people whose interest in psychosis stems from personal or family experience.

To support its aim of advancing scholarship in an inclusive and interdisciplinary way, the series benefits from the advice of an editorial board:

Katherine Berry; Sandra Bucci; Marc Calmeyn; Caroline Cupitt; Pamela Fuller; Jim Geekie; Olympia Gianfrancesco; Lee Gunn; Kelley Irmen; Sumeet Jain; Nev Jones; David Kennard; Eleanor Longden; Tanya Luhrmann; Brian Martindale; Andrew Moskowitz; Michael O'Loughlin; Jim van Os; David Shiers.

For more information about this book series visit www.routledge.com/The-International-Society-for-Psychological-and-Social-Approaches-to-Psychosis/book-series/SE0734

For more information about ISPS, email isps@isps.org or visit our website, www.isps.org.

For more information about the journal *Psychosis* visit www.isps.org/index.php/publications/journal

COMMUNITY-BASED MENTAL HEALTHCARE FOR PSYCHOSIS

From Homelessness to Recovery and Continued In-home Support

Peter Dierinck

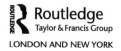

Routledge
Taylor & Francis Group

LONDON AND NEW YORK

Designed cover image: © Iryna Spodarenko as rendered as the owner of the image on Getty Images.

First published 2023
by Routledge
4 Park Square, Milton Park, Abingdon, Oxon OX14 4RN

and by Routledge
605 Third Avenue, New York, NY 10158

Routledge is an imprint of the Taylor & Francis Group, an informa business

© 2023 Peter Dierinck

The right of Peter Dierinck to be identified as author of this work has been asserted in accordance with sections 77 and 78 of the Copyright, Designs and Patents Act 1988.

British Library Cataloguing-in-Publication Data
A catalogue record for this book is available from the British Library

ISBN: 978-1-032-11464-4 (hbk)
ISBN: 978-1-032-11463-7 (pbk)
ISBN: 978-1-003-22001-5 (ebk)

DOI: 10.4324/9781003220015

Typeset in Times New Roman
by codeMantra

CONTENTS

INTRODUCTION

A Day on the Psychiatric Ward

Eight-thirty: I have had my breakfast at home, and I walk to his apartment two streets up. It is sunny and already hot. As ever, I wait longer than you normally would after ringing the bell. His voice is tentative over the inter-com: 'Peter?' 'Yes. It's me'. I have another wait coming, because the buzzer is broken and he has to come all the way down from the fourth floor to let me in. In spite of the heat, he is well wrapped up: hoodie drawn tightly about his head. It is how he likes to dress, rain or shine. He walks ahead of me and asks how I am. He will ask several times in the course of our conversation, always in the same tone as when he first greeted me. It is his way of filling in the silences. I sit down, and he asks if I would like a coffee. He made it fresh this morning; he has been expecting me, obviously. I ask if he has had breakfast. He says he hasn't. He offers me some cake and encourages me to help myself. The box is still unopened. My colleague, who has told me of her concerns about his eating so little, took him to the shop to buy a cake a few days ago. Clearly, her inducement has had no effect. I cut myself a slice in the hope that he will join me. But he doesn't. To round off my visit he and I will phone his brother, who visits regularly. Tonight his brother will bring a kebab. He loves those. He is proud to show off his television set, which was connected to the cable network yesterday. The support worker showed him how it works. He can do it. He places the two remotes by the TV set with care. It's amazing how well he concentrates at times. We go downstairs and open his mailbox. I tell him to check it once a day. And that I will make some name stickers, for his mailbox and doorbell. To make the place feel more official. He nods in satisfaction, smiles and asks if it would be difficult to make a sticker with his name on. The only letters we find are addressed to the previous tenant. We go for a walk. I show him the venue for a neigh-bourhood party this weekend. We look at the poster. It doesn't really appeal to him. But the poster mentions a community centre about a hundred yards up. A friendly man there tells us more about the place and says that you are welcome any day. It has a social grocery store, where you can collect food parcels. On Thursdays there is a free breakfast. While there, he tells me that he has been before, and that the place has a benefits office. He will repeat

DOI: 10.4324/9781003220015-1

1

this several times on the way home. It seems fairly likely that he will drop in. We walk on, and he stops outside an insurance office. A poster in the window depicts a man on a bench. He examines the poster for some time and tells me that he likes it. I gaze at it with him, aware that I have never stood before an advertising poster for so long. I don't get to hear what he likes about the poster. He tells me that he doesn't have an answer to that question. We walk on in the morning sun, and he sinks ever deeper into his own world. I hear him whisper, unintelligibly. He makes rapid up and down movements with his head, as if nodding in support of what he is telling himself. His responses to my conversation become slower and less frequent. I wonder if all these new impressions have tired him. When we come to say goodbye he is more alert. He asks again when my colleague plans to visit. I answer, he asks again and I give the same reply. It is an almost ritual repetition, which we run through again when I give him the day of my forthcoming visit. And again when I say that I will pop a letter in his mailbox with the date of his first visit from the family care services. I feel like a teacher helping a pupil to memorise a topic. As always, I am a little saddened when I leave. He is incredibly happy to be living on his own, but it takes a huge amount of energy to embrace these new experiences. By asking me things repeatedly and listening to my patient answers is he just extending our time together? Does he feel lonely at the thought of my leaving? As ever, he tells me that he does not have the answers to these questions.

Months later, this repetition of questions on parting has come to an end. Is he more familiar with independent living and his surroundings now? Or has the loneliness waned because his network has grown and more people come to visit? I suspect that both are true.

After 30 minutes, I arrive at the ward of the psychiatric centre, where I work. We have two peer supporters with us on a short training placement. They hate the term 'observation placement'. They cannot wait to get talking to the inpatients. Both are very open about their own inpatient experiences. One, Yvonne, also has much to say about her life. She has been a victim of domestic violence and was dependent on alcohol and drugs. She looks bright and alert. She is glowing. She has her difficult moments, but is feeling good now. Both peer supporters reveal a strength that will bring hope to anyone in the group who is still in inpatient care. Someone talks about the loneliness you feel when discharged from the hospital. Someone else says that there isn't enough real contact between the patients on the ward. He also says that it is great to see people coming here and talking about themselves so openly. Someone from the benefits office chimes in to say that she has been admitted to a psychiatric ward more than once in the past. She is suddenly sounding like a peer supporter herself now. Horizons are shifting. Thanks to peer supporters, the difference between healthcare professionals and patients has rapidly and significantly reduced. There is a greater sense of 'we'. And, at last, the discussion is more about exclusion and reconnection than illness and mental ill health. Just about everyone at the meeting is keen to visit the drop-in centre where the peer supporters get their training. A place where you can drop in for a coffee, or even help out in the kitchen. A place of meetings, and a place of hope.

In the afternoon we head out to a city about 13 kilometres away. I go by bike with three patients. Johan is proud that he knows the way. We avoid the traffic by cycling along a small river. He rides alongside me and, between jokes, talks about his life and his most wonderful and horrendous experiences. One of the group begins to tire, and we stop briefly to wait. We take care of each other. The sun is out, and the landscape is absolutely beautiful. We enjoy the surroundings and just being together. We are awaited by the rest of the group, who came by car. Today we are walking dogs. Kathy has brought them. They are with registered charity set up in 2008 to rescue greyhounds in need of care. The dogs were used for racing, coursing and breeding and were often kept in appalling conditions.

Ludo beams when he hears that we are walking dogs. The support workers always give Ludo the same dog, to get them used to each other, so they bond. Gavina, the dog, heads straight for Ludo. You can't drag him out of bed for anything, normally, but he wouldn't miss this for the world. He used to have a dog, he tells us, and was devastated when it died.

Michel, a local resident, has brought his own dog. Around the other dogs it seems a little excitable. Hard work for its owner, who has to keep it under control. Michel gives up in the end, reluctantly, and goes home. Our two peer support interns have joined us and are getting to know the people from this morning's group meeting.

It is quite extraordinary to see these people who are living through mental health issues smiling and walking dogs, which, like themselves, have been through terrible experiences. The lady from the charity, who is something of a dog whisperer, talks about the post-traumatic stress that some animals suffer. She really enjoys her afternoon out with the people from our centre, who take such enormous care of the animals. It does the dogs an awful lot of good. Patients talk about pets, and how important they are to them when they return to independent living. We have a quick drink on the terrace, a little chat about what we've done and then we cycle back to the centre. Fortunately, this time, we have the wind behind us.

It is a day of apparently disparate, yet not unconnected, activities. To begin with, everything revolves around care in the home rather than admission to a psychiatric hospital, and the emphasis is on the patients' own experience and their understanding of themselves. Essentially, it is about the importance of participation, which culminates in the development and deployment of expertise through lived experience. In the end, we reach beyond the peer group by establishing contact with local residents, or, that is to say, people outside the mental healthcare setting. This is the essence of quartermaking. It is about finding or creating hospitable places that are not connected to mental health services. Though different, the examples described here share a common thread.

This book argues the case for patience, compassion and perseverance in the personal relationship between healthcare professional and patient. Specifically, I would like to appeal for greater consideration for those who have lost everything and become homeless through mental ill health. It is odd that homeless people receive little or no support from mental healthcare services, and then, after entering the psychiatric system, are often seen as therapy-resistant. This is my experience. People who have lost everything through mental ill health are entitled to the appropriate help, including mental healthcare. A hospital admission can have such a stabilising effect that this in itself becomes a problem. The art is to find and develop anchorages outside the ward while the patient is still in treatment.

No child would ever dream of spending time, let alone a lifetime, in psychiatric care. As healthcare professionals, we have to put everything we have into helping people exit the psychiatric system once they enter, by giving them hope and support on the journey. For those who are homeless and sleeping in a psychiatric bed, we, our ward, find a home: for those who are seeking work, we steer a course through the maze of complex structures. As healthcare professionals, we readily admit that we do not always have the answers, but we keep searching. We never give up. We stay hopeful, in spite of the setbacks along the way.

This book also argues the case for more mental healthcare in the community. All over the world, lots of patients have spent their lives in psychiatric institutions. In 2011 the second and third highest numbers of psychiatric beds were in Belgium and the Netherlands, respectively. Only Japan has more (OECD Health Statistics, 2013). A heart-sinking conclusion. A stay on a psychiatric ward is time spent in a highly artificial environment, a world apart from a human way of life. It is best, then, that a person's long-term treatment for mental ill health is not combined with a long stay on a psychiatric ward. When treating mental ill health we should think not in terms of cure, but recovery. Discharge from a psychiatric hospital does not automatically imply an end to treatment. On the contrary. It frequently presents the ideal opportunity for treatment to begin, or resume. It is a case of trial and error for us, the coaches, and trial and error for the people we coach.

The origins of the psychiatric institution are connected to detaining people for long periods because they are not adjusted to society (Michel Foucault, *Histoire de la folie à l'âge classique*). The fact that it took away their control over their own lives was a secondary concern (Foucault, 1961). In this book, I argue the case for the patient's right to self-management. It is vital that patients be given the right to make decisions, even if in hindsight those decisions may prove to not be correct. With this approach, the healthcare process itself becomes one of trial and error. Charles E. Lindblom would call it 'muddling through' (Lindblom, 1959). We decide in small steps, look to see what happens, then decide again. It is about walking a path together, healthcare professional and patient, without knowing where it will lead. The journey does not end in the hands of any one health professional or organisation. Continuity of care implies an uninterrupted continuation of the support process.

When people find themselves in a psychiatric setting, such as a hospital, we, on our ward in the psychiatric centre in Belgium, try to give them as much control as possible and to offer the maximum potential for recovery in society by creating outlets to neighbourhood and community resources. We stay close to these patients by listening to their feelings of regret and failure, which are based on a future that was once conceived of, or even dreamt of, differently. Most of all, we are present in everything we do. Our work is based on being there. There are many aspects to being there, and, ultimately, it enables connection. For, if despondency is a mark of powerlessness, and anger leads to blame, then selfless presence can be a balm for the soul.

For anyone who is in search of figures and statistics, this book holds little interest. It gives examples, mostly, from everyday practice. Everyone is referred to by a pseudonym. Details of vignettes have been changed to ensure no one can be recognised. I have consent from everyone referred to.

I recount my own, personal journey, and refer to my many contacts: not just patients, but patient families and people and organisations outside the mental healthcare setting. On my journey, I have discovered dynamics in patients that cannot be understood through classic diagnoses, but have more to do with being human. The words used to describe a person staying in a psychiatric hospital are a matter of frequent discussion. Some, like 'resident', have a more respectful ring to them, but are not a true reflection of reality. The people we are talking about are not residents, because they do not 'reside' in the psychiatric hospital. A resident owns or rents the place he stays in. This is not true of people in psychiatric hospitals. Another term, 'services users', sounds long-winded to me. Please accept my apology if the words 'patient' and 'client', as they appear in this book, sound disrespectful. I have chosen these terms to express a relationship. I use the term 'patient' for anyone who is staying in a psychiatric hospital, and 'client' for anyone who is receiving treatment as an outpatient, usually under the care of a FACT Team. 'FACT' stands for Flexible Assertive Community Treatment. A FACT Team is a group of healthcare professionals and peer supporters who provide support at home for people with mental ill health. In other words, these terms refer to the place that a person occupies in relation to someone else.

> Sometimes I am a client, or a patient, or have a different role. It says nothing about me, but about my relationship to the person who sits opposite or cares for me. If it's a psychiatrist, I'm a patient. It makes no difference to me what I am, as long as I get the right treatment. If it's based on recovery and it gives me my autonomy, I'm happy!
> – Mirjam Giphart, peer supporter at GGZ[1]

I would like to dedicate this book to all my real-life and Facebook friends in Belgium, the Netherlands and Italy: patients, clients, family members, colleagues and community residents. I would also like to give my very special thanks to the managers of the psychiatric centres for their tireless work to improve accessibility, and for their open-mindedness, through which they not only facilitate but stimulate renewal and change.

My sincere and heartfelt thanks go also to the people in my immediate environment, who, through their fascination and dedication, and their simplicity, have revealed to me the beauty of people and, above all, life.

Parts of this book have been published previously in other forms on the internet, Socialnet and Psychosenet and in the books *Verder met kwartiermaken*, Doortje Kal, Rutger Post and Jean Pierre Wilken (eds.) and *Woonnood in Vlaanderen* (Pascal De Decker, Bruno Meeus, Isabelle Pannecoucke, Elise Schillebeeckx, Jana Verstraete, Emma Volckaert) and the magazine *Participatie en herstel* (March 2015, no. 1).

Note

1 With consent Mirjam Giphart.

References

OECD (2013), *Health at a Glance 2013: OECD Indicators*, OECD Publishing, 2013. http://dx.doi.org/10.1787/health_glance-2013-en, p. 184.

Michel Foucault, *Folie et déraison. Histoire de la folie à l'âge classique*, Paris, Gallimard, 1961.

Charles E. Lindblom, Muddling through, Science or inertia?. *Public Administration Review*, 19(2), 79–88, Spring 1959.

1

ON MODEL RAILWAYS

Looking back on my life, I can say that I have never experienced anything truly unsettling or deeply disturbing. Yes, there were moments of sadness, but they have been outweighed by the joys. The latter have come and gone with a regularity that has brought me constancy and peace of mind. But I do not think of my wonderful life as something special of my own making: I note that in the essential elements of life I have mostly been lucky. To begin with, I was lucky with the time and place of my birth. My country, Belgium, has been at peace since the day I was born. I was not born into poverty. My parents were hard working and looked after my interests. For me, they wanted a better future than they could have envisaged for themselves, and they encouraged me to study. 'Study a few years, stick at it and life will be better later on', they told me, and they were right. The mere fact that I could trust them allowed me to develop my talents to a reasonable or good effect. Other people live in poverty, or in war-torn countries. Or their parents were less trustworthy, so they received poor advice as children or, worse still, none at all. In the fundamentals of life, many people have been short of luck or had none at all. Some were left to fend for themselves, even abused, by their parents. I cannot take the credit for the parents I was born to. I was lucky. When you recognise that pride has no place in how you turn out, because how you turn out has very little to do with you, then you realise that you need not feel shame if the results are disappointing. I hold onto this thought when I meet people to whom life has been less kind, as I do throughout my work as a psychologist. It gives me a sense of compassion for those whose fate is different from mine.

I examine and re-examine my life's events, and, when I do, I explore different interpretations for my own actions and others' actions towards me. At times I find the coherence I was looking for, at others I do not. It is a journey with which I think we are all familiar. We try to eliminate the very contradictions that make us human. We do not always stick to our original intentions, and we sometimes do things we did not want to and later regret. After the facts, we look for reasons, excuses and theories to explain our

DOI: 10.4324/9781003220015-2

behaviour, so we see ourselves as the people we want to be and move on with our lives. I compare this search, this writing of an autobiography, to a child piecing together a model railway. Like the child, I will use long, straight sections of track wherever I can, with the fewest possible bends and even fewer switches. Only if absolutely necessary, and to keep the train moving, will I use branches and sidings. On the railway, built by this method, my train of thoughts is free to travel unhindered, from the first stop to the last, looking back on my life. From beginning to present day. Significant events I barely remember, wild behavioural contradictions, events I would rather forget, moments of confusion and upheaval: these are the furnishings in the room where our child lays the tracks. They are the tables and chairs, the walls and the rough ground that stand in the way. They are the obstacles to be overcome as I lay down the tracks of my memory, my story.

I smooth out the rough terrain by tracing cause and effect, to make sense of events that at first seemed coincidental. I flatten the surface by laying roadbeds to level the tracks. I build bridges across ravines – events that tore my life apart – reconnecting banks as if they were never disconnected. The construction work is often difficult, uncomfortable and downright painful, but sorely needed. The train must roll on. It is not in its nature to stop. The tracks of my memory are repaired and the train travels without issue, without stopping. As a precaution, I slow it down in these places. Here, I know the track is less stable. I build as solidly as I can, but leave room for replacements and more switches in the future. The ground I cover is prone to landslides and subsidence. Patches, covering gaps in my story, may no longer be adequate. Repairs, initially effective, may suddenly fail, and tracks may be in need of re-alteration. It is a never-ending task.

Like permanent scars, the bridges and roadbeds mark the sites of previously spanned chasms. It is here that most of the repairs are done to strengthen the tracks and let the train pass unhindered. They are the weakest points on the route, in need of regular maintenance, regular rituals for my sorrow and grief. Also to be commemorated are the anniversaries of life-disrupting events. Rituals that may be needed for a lifetime. They are an essential part of our existence. Our life, our permanent recovery project.

People who have spent time in a psychiatric hospital also seek explanations for cause and effect. What happened to me? How did I arrive on a psychiatric ward? How do I mend the ruptures in my life, the rips left by psychosis? Why did I do what I've done? Why have I misused drugs? Some of these questions, like 'why did my father abuse me?' are extremely difficult to bridge. They reveal an irreparable breach in the network, where the train comes to a halt. People search for meaning in past events, to help them proceed with their lives. Recovery is about creating a meaningful life. (Deegan and Stracker, 2004, p. 11) It can be done with words and language, but, where none is available, by finding a place or activity that links to a deeply buried desire. It is usually a combination of the two.

Much of what I do as a psychologist is work on these ideas with people, on this journey. Help them lay their own model railway. For them, the solutions rarely come in straight sections, but rely on a mass of bends and switches. Work on their railway is often difficult, and we end up searching for that one particular switch for a given place in the network. A switch that does not come as standard; that has to be made, 'custom'-made. It is about finding the switch that gets you around the obstacle, gets the train rolling again. Creating that custom-made switch usually involves more than just reflecting on your life: it involves what I describe in this book as *quartermaking.*

> After decades of hospital admissions John finds the courage to re-vocalise his old desire to be a teacher, get married and have children. Early in his admissions he would mention it frequently, but as time went on he stopped. Health professionals grew tired of hearing it, and, since they stopped listening, he thought it unimportant himself. The old desire was deeply buried; even he had forgotten it. Now, he rarely speaks at all. All he does is move. He seems to be fleeing from his previous life. One colossal disaster that flashes past repeatedly like a bolt of lightning. He moves so as not be moved and flees from one institution to another. It is a search for peace. He can no longer connect to the desire, which is now lost to his consciousness, and so life has no meaning.

To express this unfulfilled desire is to work on recovery. But it terrifies him to express it. We are not looking for a switch based on language, or speech, but creating a custom-made switch to restore life's meaning. We do this through quartermaking: the creation of welcoming places. The patient perspective in general is nicely illustrated in a quote that is attributed to Albert Einstein: 'You do not have to understand the world, you just have to find your own way around in it.' By burying his desires he has become isolated, he has descended deeper into the psychiatric treatments that brought his train to a standstill. The switch is literally a new and different territory, where he wants to go and live. A place far from the scene of the disaster. Quartermaking is the means by which we attempt to prepare a new territory for a new resident.

People recover, and so do places: so do cities, and villages. A while ago, when pondering the introduction for a lecture I was giving in Ypres, it seemed obvious to call the place a city in recovery. Ypres was on the western front in the First World War. It was utterly obliterated, and the British, who lost many lives there, wanted it to stay that way. The ruins would serve as a permanent reminder of the horrors that had taken place (Dendooven and De Wilde, 2020). But the people of Ypres wanted their city back. They wanted it to have a future, not just a past. Not the open wound of these ruins. Nor did they want to pretend that the trauma, the many fallen, the utter destruction of the mediaeval centre, had never occurred. So the city was rebuilt as it had stood before the war, and places of remembrance were constructed. One of those is the Menin Gate, where, a hundred years after the war, the Last Post is still played every evening to remember the dead. Life in the city goes on, but the many war cemeteries stretch across the region like scars. They are places where people go to remember. Recovery is about building a meaningful life, while at the same time remembering and commemorating the constraints, the traumas. It is by looking to the past from the present that a future becomes possible. The great thing about Ypres is that it uses the war and the destruction to show itself to the world as a city of peace. This positive message cuts through the war and suffering and is received as a message of hope, a way to a better future. It is through peace, the opposite face to war, that the city conveys this message so well. It is poised between allowing life to go on and commemorating the terrible events of over a century ago. Ritual has mended the rips and tears that were once inflicted on this city. Ypres is now a symbol of peace for the world. A city of hope.

In my own recovery project (the alignment of my past, present and future) the model railway begins at the point furthest from me. Though hazy and illusive, these cherished early memories provide good sturdy rails and a solid base for the network. When the train leaves the station, rolling over those early memory tracks, I know that it is off to a good start, free to gather speed and cover ground without mishap.

The very first sections of track, the memory tracks, are built on two memories, very early memories, of a woman. I am not entirely sure if she is the same person in both, but I think she is. Or, to make my story complete, I hope she is. This woman is extraordinary. Her behaviour is unlike anything that I, as a child, have come to associate with adult women.

My bedroom, in my parents' house. I am a child. It is a summer's day. I am so sick in bed that all I can do is concentrate on the wallpaper pattern. I know the patterns so well that I stare at them to feel better. The fever persists. I turn my head and I see, pressed to the window, the face of a woman I do not recognise. Hands cupped around her eyes, to gaze in past the reflection of her face. At first I think the fever is giving me hallucinations, but when I close and reopen my eyes the face is still there. Afraid, I begin to shout and cry. To reach my window, she must have come in off the street and walked across our garden.

Mother rushes in and sees the woman there. She seems to know her, calls her by name and waves her away. The woman takes to her heels. She is genuinely startled at my mother's displeasure. Mother explains that the lady is a little simple-minded but means no harm. There is no need to be afraid, she is a nice lady.

When the fear ebbs away, I am left with shame at having been afraid and regret at having allowed the woman to be chased away. I have never forgotten the incident, and I am thankful to my parents for having the decency to tell me that not everyone who behaves a little strangely or oddly is necessarily dangerous. For a long time, I daydream about seeing her at my window again, even starting a conversation with her. Nothing special, just about the weather or something, or saying that I was sick, that I'd had the flu when she first appeared at my window and that that was why I had been given such a start.

It is the early 1970s. I must be about 12. I am with my parents and my brother at a fair on the outskirts of the village. We hear a marching band approach. A drum roll. People step aside. I move a little closer to the shooting gallery. A few metres in front of the majorettes, who are in full costume, parades a woman in vintage work clothes. She looks dirty and unkempt but is dancing, laughing out loud, turning her head from side to side and waving her arms about wildly. When the music stops and the majorettes and players pause, she puts on her serious face. She keeps the beat, and checks behind for when the others start to move again. When they do, she dances on with the same enthusiasm, maintaining the illusion that it is she, arms waving for her entourage, who sets the tempo. Onlookers applaud and laugh at her antics. She is stealing the show and boy does she know it. She does not seem to care whether people are laughing at her or with her. It's carnival time, and she's making the most of it. I ask my mother what is wrong with the woman, why she is doing this. Mother looks slightly surprised at how clueless I am. It is the first time I have seen anyone behave so out of the ordinary. The straightforwardness with which the bystanders watch her, without fear, puts me at ease and gives this odd spectacle a sense of familiarity and safety. My fascination and awe at those who behave a little oddly, but live in the community, stays with me as of then.

A third and very brief memory. My parents, my brother and I drive past an entranceway that stretches back and disappears into the gloom. I peer briefly into the darkness, at which point my mother says that we are passing the 'loony bin'. The word sounds so laden to me now, but she utters it in a hushed and serious tone that expresses respect, even reverence. She can't tell me exactly who lives there, and her lack of an answer only deepens the mystery in my mind. I determine to go sometime, to see what it looks like and find out who lives there. The memory has a photographic quality about it now: a wide drive, an illuminated entrance, all else in darkness.

Later, I hear my parents say that a great aunt, one of my grandfather's sisters, had been committed to that institution for a very long time; thirty years or so. My relatives came in pairs; only my great uncle in-law was alone, without a partner. That seemed very odd to me, and it made me curious. The family never spoke of his wife. Or at least only rarely, and tentatively. And awkward pauses and silences would ensue if I asked too many questions.

If she was mentioned it would be in relation to her deep distrust, which could lead to aggressive outbursts towards her husband, my great uncle. I heard compassion in the family's voices, deep compassion, and respectful amazement at the strangeness of the human mind. I realised how difficult this was for my relatives to talk about, not just because they found it inexplicable, but because it hurt, it was shameful. And in the presence of my great uncle she was never mentioned at all.

To me, my fascination with this woman related to things unseen and unspoken. I came no closer to seeing my great uncle's wife than to seeing her peers on that gloomy evening, as we passed the 'loony bin'. They lived apart, in large buildings, at the end of drives so long that you couldn't see them from the street. Far from everything and everyone else. To me, psychiatric institutions were secluded places, where people who did odd things would stay, not for fun, or for their own good, but through necessity, for being who they were. All you could do was pity them with a shake of your head and hope that you didn't end up the same way. 'There's nowt stranger than folk', as my mother would say. She was always a little rueful when she said it, conscious that it was equally applicable to her.

The following memory is much clearer in my mind. In secondary school, I give a talk on a book about psychiatry. *Kleine psychiatrie* by a Dutch professor (Van den berg, 1966). It is one of the first books I buy. I still have a copy, in my library. At that time, the mid-1970s, I am fascinated by its photographs, especially of the people shown in strange positions in bed. Courtesy of this book I get my first glimpse of these people, always hidden to me before. I can still see them now. I list the illnesses in my talk and show the accompanying pictures by way of illustration. Above a caption that reads 'depressive phase of manic-depressive psychosis; image of distressed state' there is a photograph of what looks like a Surinamese woman in a nightgown, her face contorted in distress. On the opposite page, a photograph of the same woman, fully dressed, smiling slightly, with below it a caption saying: 'same patient as in previous photograph; hypomanic state immediately after depressive phase, shortly before recovery'. The photographs appear to have been included as a visual teaching aid, like a map for a geography lesson, and this is how I use them in my talk. I have inserted markers to make it easy for me to find the photographs while reading. The teacher likes the talk but criticises my use of the photographs. He says you could ask anyone off the street to pull a face, then photograph it to illustrate the text. He thinks that photographs illustrating the illnesses add nothing to my talk. I have never forgotten this feedback. A person's face can tell you a lot about their emotional state but does not necessarily say anything about their mental health. So the hidden people in my mind looked not so very different from me. And so, by extension, they were not so very different from me. I remember being slightly disappointed at this discovery. I had been looking for the mystery and excitement in the other, the anomalous. But there was still the question as to why these people, if they weren't so very different, were forced to stay in those buildings. And what actually went on there? Who worked there? What special abilities were needed to deal with these people? After the talk I was no closer to knowing. It felt like I was on the periphery again, not seeing people, not knowing anything about them.

Later I thought that this fascination with the slightly odd, this standing on the periphery, had as much to do with me. At parties, I always wanted to be the DJ, not just one of the revellers. The DJ was out on the edge, in some respects, but vital to setting a party mood: yet another aspect of my own character.

The photos I had discovered in *Kleine psychiatrie* (Van den berg, 1966) continued to influence my thoughts on psychiatry. I am ashamed to admit it, but when I started my first psychology placement, in an inpatient ward in 1986, I still thought that many of the patients would be treated in their beds.

Though almost 30 years have passed, I remember that placement vividly. I was introverted and had very little contact with the staff; all the more time, then, for the patients on the ward. I was with them often, had no office of my own and always spoke with patients in 'between times' when there was no therapy. Patients were not all that keen on therapy in general, and I, as the intern, was asked to encourage them to go. The therapy rooms were across the road. So I spent a lot of time walking patients there. In many cases, it was the chance to walk alongside them rather than the therapy, that prompted them to come. I realised then that people with mental ill health were often quite happy in my company, as I had a way of listening and relating to them. I heard them say I was a good listener. Those informal moments were excellent for establishing real connections. The patients tended to act a little differently in therapy. With me they were casual and spontaneous. I did not take therapy sessions or do official interviews, so I found myself in *their time*. Back then, it was plain to me that everyday life of people was far more important than therapy time. So they needed support in the everyday life. When I was on placement I loved communal life on the ward. Some patients would stay in their rooms, to be alone, and others would occupy the same seat in the common room, day after day. They would stare silently into space, and seemed to wait for dinner-time, medicine-time or bedtime as a cue to move. These moments were like monastery prayer times. Dividers to mark out the day. In an institution like this, time could be an issue. When there is too much time to kill, points that subdivide the time, like bedtime and meal times, are incredibly helpful.

In those days I thought that coexisting in a building like a psychiatric institution automatically created a bond between the people who lived there, precisely because they lived there together. I thought they saw themselves as a group and felt that they had something in common. I thought that being together in isolation from the rest of society created a sense of community, a warmth, and I wanted to experience it. Soak it up. I thought that the people I accompanied to therapy, a group of six, believed they had something in common, and that this belief created solidarity. And yet, at the times when this seemed most apparent to me, I was forgetting my own influence. Although they cared for each other because they wanted to, they often did so because I cared for them. I was not aware that patients might loath each other purely because they had ended up in the same wretched situation. One marginalised person might view another with a mixture of pity and anger, because in the other he/she recognised their own wretchedness. At times it would be those who shunned the group, especially on walks outside the institution, who fought hardest to escape this place of isolation. They would have nothing to do with the people inside the institution, because they still identified with the people outside.

> I will never forget Linda, who was going to knit me a jumper and made a beautiful ceramic figurine for me. She had a friend on the ward, a feisty woman, who spoke cynically about the world outside the institution, yet showered her companions with compliments and gifts. She would draw people to her in the common room, and it was always fun. After leaving the ward Linda never came to visit, which deeply saddened her friend. She could gather people around in a psychiatric setting, but not outside the institution. She couldn't understand why her friend, now discharged, never came to visit. In those days my sympathies lay with the lady who made life fun. Later, much later, my sympathies lay with Linda.

Besides patients, I would see healthcare professionals in the *between time*, which was also my time. They were competent ward nurses and good therapists, who could be found in their own rooms. I would stay on for a chat after therapy sessions. The therapists were more likely to share their dreams and frustrations. They frequently felt constrained by the endless regulations involved in running a large organisation. They were creative, and they planted seeds that got me thinking outside the box.

I was placed on the admissions ward, which occupied two floors. Downstairs was more expensive. It was where the less troubled people stayed. Piano in the common room, red velvet on the chairs. Plush carpets over the creaky parquet. As you entered through the decorated glass door you would be watched by more elderly women, seated stiffly and quite uncomfortably on the old chairs. It looked like a once luxurious but now jaded waiting room. Most of the time it was eerily quiet in there. You could feel the seconds ticking by. It had to be quiet, because the people were here for rest. The silence actually got on my nerves. Upstairs was where the slightly poorer, people stayed. It was noisier. You heard laughter and raised voices. People hardly ever stayed in their seats. It had atmosphere. I liked it better upstairs.

I saw monks who stopped patients taking food to their rooms at meal-times and were ready to pick a fight with any patient who tried. I saw psychiatrists in white coats, with stethoscopes, approach and sit beside patients in the common room, to check their blood pressure. They were exerting their authority. After a blood-pressure measurement, they would block any further conversation with patronising and conciliatory words to the effect that everything would be fine, and then they would hurry off.

In team meetings, the same doctors lectured nurses who would never, in their wildest dreams, have considered contradicting a psychiatrist. Once, on placement, when I questioned a patient's diagnosis, everyone in the room fell silent and waited anxiously for what would happen next. It was the doctor who had the final word. I heard later that the psychiatrist had been unappreciative, to say the least, of my attempted dialogue. Nothing was ever said about it to me.

I have never forgotten how important it is to place the patient and their healthcare on a level and to connect with a patient, or how important the informality of the *between time* actually is: a chat on the terrace, in the corridor, at the kitchen sink, after the morning meeting, before leaving for home... I still leave my door open between appointments regularly, so that patients can come for an informal chat, often through the open door. In that sense, I am still a little student-like in the way I go about things, as well as in the sense that I have an awful lot to learn, especially from those who have seen it all and done it all before.

I completed my placement there, got a job as a psychologist there and went on to become a conscientious objector. It was the late 1980s, when group therapies were hailed as the answer to everything. A balanced regime of talking therapies and activity therapies was applied. We wrote weekly schedules: patients had to cook, wash up, tidy their rooms and clean the corridors. They were expected to work on creative activities, sports and social skills. Everything was compulsory, for we were certain that we had unlocked the path to a cure. Take part and you would get better, of that we had no doubt. *We* knew what was best for *them*. All that remained, or so it seemed, was to convince the patients of this. To our surprise, however, the patients were not all that impressed with our recipe for success. I gave classes in social skills. All kinds of social interactions were served up through videotaped examples. Week after week I introduced a new set of social skills to a group of people who were at times feeling so psychotic that they could hardly summon the concentration to follow. Few were genuinely interested. Some of the more outspoken participants complained that it felt like boot camp. The friendlier ones said it reminded them of school. And, for most of them, school had been a very negative experience. Later, I stopped giving classes in social skills.

I am even more ashamed to say that permission for weekend leave would occasionally rest on having attended enough of those therapy sessions. I did

15

not feel good in this system. It was so different from what I experienced in my earliest memories, when I was very interested in these people without the longing to change them.

In this system, we were at a place where people had to be readied for a return to society, a society based on power and achievement. And we, the healthcare professionals, were convinced of our ability to deliver. I remember the growing doubts and concerns. We had a feeling that something wasn't right. If a person was capable of living independently and could afford to eat in a social restaurant, a place where poor people eat at reduced price, why force cooking lessons on them in the run-up to their discharge? The staff began to discuss these issues. We tried to be more considerate of the patients' own wishes, not those of the organisation. And we paid greater attention to each person's immediate environment. Compulsory attendance of therapies was questioned. It was a tough and difficult battle in the team at times, and I left. With a heavy heart, I parted ways with some very creative colleagues. I have kept in touch with many for a very long time, and we always get along well when we meet.

In the early 1990s I had a new employer, another psychiatric centre. I opted for a rehabilitation ward. At the time, many colleagues saw this as a strange choice. We were at the peak of an era that was all about treating and changing people. Congresses and workshops in Belgium made no mention of rehabilitation. The word recovery was not used then, but it had already been by the early proponents like Pat Deegan and by the survivor movement. Patients were described as 'untreatable' (Petry, 2011). Those patients were kept on the oldest wards. The ones last in line for 'alteration and renovation'. My ward contained patients that had been referred to a so-called 'longer stay' ward after a string of treatment failures, and had fallen deeper into the net of psychiatry, further from the front door, the place nearest society: the admissions ward. I use the word 'net' because it was assumed they would never escape the psychiatric system; an assumption that was often borne out. They had been abandoned. Well, this was where I thought I could make a difference. These were the people I could really get behind. I wanted to do something for the abandoned, those for whom regimes had not been developed. A position I have always maintained.

In those days, wards in Belgium would identify a group and then develop a group therapy programme. They applied strict selection procedures based on intakes. So strict, in fact, that they preferred empty beds over people that did not match the profile. Much was made of the diagnosis, to be certain that the right patient arrived in the right place, on the right regime. Organisational thinking. Pigeon holes waiting for people to fill them. Caregivers were searching for patients who they thought had the best chance of recovery. The knowledge lay with the therapists. And they could be non-communicative with any patient who queried a diagnosis. Diagnosis was the preserve of the healthcare professional.

Most of what I had seen in previous years had been organisational think-ing: division into observation groups, treatment groups, resocialisation groups. Each group had a regime in keeping with its identity. Some health professionals thought that patients would only succeed if they completed the regime and earned their discharge.

I wanted to get away from set regimens and standard regimes. Where better to start than with the very people who had been failed by regimens and regimes?

It seemed to me that the existing care was designed around people with good verbal skills, the capacity to reflect on their lives and, frequently, a middle-class background. But for those who were experiencing severe psychosis, people with moderate learning difficulties, those with therapy fatigue, people who did not see the point of talking about their problems, there were no remedies, no methods. These people were often left with a very long stay in the institution with no prospect of ever coming out (Petry, 2011). It was my ambition to work with these very people. I stood by those who had been sentenced to remain in the psychiatric system, not by their own choosing, but through a lack of support. What they needed was a vision based on social exclusion, and a method by which to oppose that exclu-sion. Among the healthcare professionals on this ward, there were some who could no longer cope elsewhere. It was a landing place for nurses, psycholo-gists and psychiatrists. They came from the more 'acute' wards and had been transferred, some at their own request, to these 'quiet' wards, where little was expected of them, or little more than was expected of the patients transferred there. Some did manage to see out their careers in comfort on these wards, but it was here, remarkably enough, that a few others discov-ered a new lease of life. They were wonderful co-workers and colleagues, and we worked together for many years.

A few others, who were not happy with their transfer to the rehab ward, resented having to work with patients labelled untreatable. They failed either to understand or recognise the value of this shift from patient to citizen. They reasoned that they, like their colleagues, had every right to work with patients who could be expected to 'see results'. The ones that were referred to our ward because they were no longer proficient on another ward saw in these untreatable patients a reflection of their own incompetence, which they preferred to ignore by refusing to admit patients or re-referring them to even longer-stay wards as soon as they were able. These dissatisfied health-care professionals did not wish to see 'untreatable' patients on the ward. This gave rise to discussions about which profiles the ward should target.

In the end we wondered: why not specialise in people who fall through the net? Why not develop 'expertise' around them, with their help? We surmised that they would have something to teach us. They might show us something hitherto unnoticed in the healthcare profession. I, along with a few like-minded people on the team, was prepared to forego our existing knowledge, which was largely based on more easily treatable, and often middle-class patients. But would I really have to jettison everything I had learned? Or just parts, and if so, which ones? To begin with, we decided not to operate a low-access intake procedure on the ward, and this gave us a highly varied population. We would exclude no one who was referred to us. As a psychologist, I was trained to help people gain an insight into their behaviour, so they could alter it and have a better life. Well, not necessarily better. Insight is the important thing. In training, I learned that the patients themselves had to discover what had gone wrong, and that I could give feedback. As a healthcare professional, the most important thing I could do was stick to the sidelines and not allow my own desires too much influence.

Recovery and quartermaking are part and parcel of the rehabilitation idea, which can also be seen as a 'restoration of honour', the right to live outside the psychiatric institution, but it was not until later, by my own doing, that they became policy on the ward.

On the subject of rehabilitation, I later heard that long-stay patients should be given the chance to function effectively in as near-to-normal a situation as possible (Bennett in Wing, 1978) and Shepherd (1984). Rehabilitation was supposed to maximise client functioning. But all that seemed inadequate to me when I listened to the grievances of those who had been admitted to the ward. They wanted to belong to society. They wanted to participate, and they wanted to do so without needing or wanting to change. This 'as near-to-normal a situation as possible' was not viable. Soon after discharge, those patients were often readmitted. They appeared to be stuck in an institution, on a psychiatric ward.

The patients in the psychiatric centre's rehab ward spoke mostly of rejection and exclusion. Many seemed deeply depressed. I often heard about thoughts of suicide. More than 90 percent were homeless. Did I just have to make them see that self-pity was hampering their reintegration? Would it then be enough to work on their self-esteem, to enable them to cope with life again? And, if that were satisfactorily achieved, would they automatically build a new life in as near-to-normal a situation as possible? Before commencing this work I wanted to see how real their stories of exclusion were. Perhaps they truly were excluded.

I tried it out for myself first. I visited estate agents with them, looking for a place to rent. I got a slightly commiserating look from the assistant, who asked me why, if I was so confident in my clients' ability to pay the rent, I did not put up the bond myself? At another agency, they gave me a friendly low-down on how the system actually works: landlords place people who are on benefits, have mental health issues on top of that, and live in an institution, at the very bottom of the 'ideal tenants' list. I accompanied patients on their search for voluntary work. That was not simple either. The patients I accompanied to clubs and associations to sign up for meaningful recreational activities were often refused.

I found that much of what people were telling me was based in reality. Their depression was not necessarily due to illness. Their despondency ensued from the slim chance of ever finding a gratifying or reassuring exit from the ward. They felt that they had become dependent on healthcare professionals, who made them do pointless therapies.

When I really listened to these people, by going out and about with them, it was not they, but I, who developed insight. I stopped seeing their reality as a subjective experience that I would have to change. My training had taught me about the dynamics of the subconscious, but now I was instead seeing societal mechanisms at work. I learnt all about power relations and social exclusion. I discovered that psychologists and psychiatrists often ascribe a patient's problems to his/her state of mind, when the true causes are rooted in society. Rather than change these societal relations, psychologists and psychiatrists altered the patient's experience, with or without medication, and contributed unwittingly, and unwillingly, to the preservation of these relational inequalities. I wondered why some people gravitated to the psychiatric system whereas others, with equally or more severe issues, did not. I discovered that integration was possible only with give and take, and that people who had been admitted for psychiatric care were viewed as having nothing more to give. I wondered what I could do to give them another opportunity to show that they could still be of meaning to others outside the institution. Long before FACT Teams (Flexible assertive community treatment teams that provide long-term care for people with severe mental illness who are not in psychiatric hospitals) appeared in Flanders our team had in 1997 set up a home care service to strengthen our hand in negotiations with landlords. This was because landlords were more inclined to rent accommodation to our clients when we offered 'home support'. I found a way to negotiate with the letting agents. I discovered that healthcare providers could establish close links with clubs and associations, making them more likely to welcome the people I was helping into the fold. I was heartened by the task that lay before me. The rehab team gradually shifted its focus to this work, and we developed expertise. Instead of providing healthcare, we were *providing hope*.

I had made the transition. I was listening to people who were no longer patients to me, but, above all, lived-experience experts and citizens. I learnt the term 'recovery' fairly late in the process. But, at the point of transition, 2012, I abandoned much of what I had learned and threw in my lot with the notion of recovery (Ostrow and Adams, 2012).

My beginning and my end, my earliest memories and my current work, were now aligned. I had come full circle. I had rediscovered my childlike sense of awe and the fear I had felt at the odd behaviour of a person I had encountered in my seemingly normal world. A journey that I had embarked on to make people better had ended up giving me a socially responsible attitude to exclusion and inclusion. I see exclusion as an injustice to be eliminated.

My work relates closely to who I am, what I aim to do and what I find important in life. I have what I consider to be a very meaningful existence. I want to connect people. The railway of memories, along which the train of consciousness passes, appears to be circular: its start and end points are connected. The ground between beginning and end – the story I have recounted above – seems to have been a necessary detour. Without it, I would have been running on the spot. To come full circle means to depart: or there can be no return. To arrive where you started is to arrive at a place that merely seems unchanged. The detour is the journey of experience and adventure, and that you have been enriched by your arrival back at the start. In that sense, I cherish the detour. The beginning – my early memories of the odd lady from my childhood – is deeply connected to the end – my current understanding of my work. That strange woman from my childhood felt connected to the community she lived in. She was not feared. People thought her odd, but welcomed her oddness and accepted it with compassion. She had a place in the community and it made her happy. She was not removed, hidden away in a huge building, far from everyone else, but allowed the chance to be seen in the community that I was a part of.

In all that I do today, I am amazed by those who stand firm in a society that demands much but gives little in return. I am in awe of those who may appear a little odd but are not forced to sacrifice that oddness to find their place. Through this sense of awe I help them regain or improve their social situation, despite, or at times thanks to, that very difference.

In the chapters that follow I discuss recovery and quartermaking: the essence of mental healthcare in the community.

References

Bennett D.H., Social forms of psychiatric treatment. In J.K. Wing (ed.), *Schizophrenia: Towards a new synthesis*, London, Academic Press, pp. 211–231, 1978.

Pat Deegan and Terry Stracker, *Building a meaningful life after hospital*, DVD-video, Center for Mental Health Services [Washington, D.C.] en 2006, ©2004.

Dominiek Dendooven and Jan De Wilde, *De wederopbouw in Ieper!*, Ieper, Flanders Fields Museum, 2020.

Laysha Ostrow and Neal Adams, Recovery in the USA: From politics to peer support. *International Review of Psychiatry*, 24(1), 70–78, 2012.

Detlev Petry, *Uitbehandeld maar niet opgegeven*, Amsterdam, Ambo, 2011.

G. Shepherd, *Institutional care and rehabilitation*, London, Longman 1984.

Prof J.H. Van den berg, *Kleine psychiatrie*, Nijkerk, Callenbach, 1966.

2

HOMELESS AND IN MENTAL
ILL HEALTH

2.1 The Experience of Space

He has torn free of the rules and obligations and discovered absolute freedom. The world now lies at his feet. So goes the romantic notion of the homeless person, the rough sleeper. A romantic fantasy cherished by those who spend a lifetime amassing it all – a house, garden, job, friends – and then, through tedium, wish to throw it away and start again. The odd dreamer indulges in the fantasy, has time out and goes on a world tour.

Homelessness is a feature of all ages and cultures. But it would be inhumane to downplay the endless misery of homelessness and make our peace with it. So intolerable is homelessness that we must keep grappling with the issue on behalf of homeless people. It represents a very deep separation from the community and generates an intense emotional response. The feeling of not being wanted burns with a barely supportable intensity.

The rough sleeper, the homeless person, is almost symbolic of loss itself. It was not by choice. All was not sacrificed for freedom. All was lost.

Through my contact in Belgium with street outreach workers, the people who do the most for this group, I know that the majority of homeless people have mental health issues (Balasuriya, Buelt, and Tsai, 2020).

It is often because of these issues that they no longer have a home. Neglected or poorly maintained properties and problems with neighbours or money force many onto the streets.

Worst of all, healthcare services do not see many of the homeless people with mental health issues as help seekers, because they may not make requests for support. Building on the work of Andries Baart, Doortje Kal writes:

> (free translation) The core of the problem is that the help-seeker 'is still to become' the help requester in the process. Acknowledgement is the core value (...) it helps if in the meeting with the professional the person concerned does not have to cut his or her problem to a size that suits the institution (...) The fact that the client does not

DOI: 10.4324/9781003220015-3

open his mail (frightened as he is of the content), does not attend his appointments (through absent-mindedness or fear of what is to come), does not keep his paperwork in order, or is not to the point, must be understood in its context (...) the logic of the client counts.

(Baart, 2001)

Baart states that there should be no question of guilt.

Once a person ends up on the streets the road out is arduous. Without money or a home, a new dynamic, that of scarcity, produces an even greater vulnerability. This dynamic is described with absolute clarity in *Scarcity. Why having too little means so much* (Mulainathan and Shafir, 2013). Scarcity has exactly the same effect on everyone, whether they are clever or stupid, thin-skinned or thick-skinned. The worse the circumstances, and the harder it becomes to find money, or friends, for example... the more a person's thoughts and actions change. More than a cramp on resources, scarcity produces a mindset, a kind of tunnel vision. We each have a given mental capacity or bandwidth. Scarcity narrows that bandwidth. When you do not know if you will eat today, the thought occupies your mind, making you unable to consider anything else. Forced into short-term thinking, you lose sight of the long-term goals. It is a matter of survival: borrowing, stealing, dodging bus and tram fares, and so on. These are all means of survival in the short term, but in the long term they imply high-interest repayments, fines, jail time... This short-term mentality, a result of homelessness and poverty, is extremely difficult to cast off. You need someone to help you in the short term, but in a way that leaves you with spare bandwidth or the mental capacity for long-term thinking. While short-term solutions, such as night shelters for the homeless, are very good, they are not enough to escape the problem in the long term. Formal carers must be aware of this and willing to think in the long term, even if this is not one of the pressing concerns of the person in their care.

> He was involuntarily admitted and assigned an administrator. These measures were designed to help and support him. But he finds it all extremely restrictive. His allowance isn't quite enough. He doesn't buy a ticket on the bus, and the fines pile up, because, as he sees it, the administrator pays. It is as if he no longer views the money, managed by the administrator on his behalf, as his own. He was arrested several years ago and held in a cell until his administrator paid the soaring fines. He never stays in the same hospital for long, so never takes the time to find decent rental accommodation. He ends up taking a room with a slum landlord. With no tenancy agreement to sign, he doesn't need the administrator's consent. A solution that works well in the short term. The room is tiny, overpriced, poorly appointed. He gets into an argument with

the landlord and finds himself on the street overnight. He roams around in a suicidal state and is involuntarily admitted. He has lost his home, now his freedom, and it weighs heavily on him. He felt so severely restricted that there was no room in his mind for long-term planning, and he seized on solutions that seemed, briefly, to advance his situation but in reality only increased his vulnerability. This administration of his affairs does not get him thinking in the long-term. The sense of scarcity does not take him beyond thoughts of the immediate future.

We write up a list of decisions, in order of priority. His involuntary detainment causes him the most trouble, so we start by lifting it. We take the risk that he won't run away, roam the streets, become suicidal again, And, now that we have won his trust, he stays to work on the following objectives. We ask the administrator for extra money for clothing and a computer. He feels like he owns something again. After losing everything he seemed unable to attach. When we assume a few of the administrative tasks, such as applying for a free bus pass, his mental capacity increases. This stops the fines heaping up in the long term. We recognise that, in the very long term, he would like to be rid of his administrator, but first we will find him a home. We also arrange home counselling. We help set up the contacts, so he feels like progress is being made. With every positive result he gains the courage to look further ahead. We help him with calls to authorities, write letters of referral, arrange intakes and look into rental accommodation with him... We update him on every new step we have taken, and we reiterate what the future steps will be. When he is down in the dumps about waiting lists, repeated form filling and doing intake interviews, we remind him constantly of the steps already taken, to turn his attention to the progress made. We link short-term and long-term thinking by establishing a list of priority interventions. With our help he gets a few minor results, which encourage him to look further ahead, beyond the day itself.

We arrange a team meeting in the meantime, attended by friends and healthcare professionals, which he finds supportive. His friends and healthcare professionals are informed of the goals and plans, and assured that we are going for continuity in his care by helping him reach his goals. It was he who selected the people at this meeting, so we can be certain of the support they are giving him. It seems more like a meeting of friends, although some of the participants are healthcare professionals he knows from before.

Homelessness is one of the most extreme consequences of mental ill health. After losing a home, people with mental ill health experience an added vulnerability, which sometimes covers or camouflages their original mental health problems. It becomes impossible to tell which came first: the mental health problem or the homelessness. In the end, unravelling the actual cause and effect is of little help. The majority of homeless people have mental health issues. Very often they have had traumatic childhood experiences, as a result of which they carry the brand of homelessness, a mark that will reveal itself time and again (Boudewijnstichting, 2022). The severity of the trauma is such that they are not really served by ordinary healthcare services (Bloemink, 2016). Many homeless people with mental health issues are no longer welcome at psychiatric institutions, and appropriate long-term help does not exist on the streets.

Homelessness often evokes all kinds of contradictory feelings in the bystander, such as revulsion, powerlessness, pity, aversion, fear and insecurity, just as insanity can do.

> (free translation) Many welfare institutions openly tell many of them that there is little or nothing more that they can do. This also means that there is no hierarchy of interventions through which these people can achieve good in the rest of their lives. The biographies are conserved in their misery as it were. The social horizon is usually obscured and many healthcare providers, as expert and concerned actors, tend to be spectators, hi-jacked as it were by unceasing chaotic events that defy reasonable interpretation and control.
>
> (Marius Nuy, *De nacht van Nederland*, p. 65)

The homeless are seen by a lot of caregivers working in psychiatric hospitals as people for whom nothing more can be done. Present-day mental healthcare is based on a request for support, which can be defined as faithful attendance at appointments. People with mental ill health do not see the appointments themselves as supportive, because they feel mistrust for society in general and so also for caregivers Therefore, the help on offer may be highly conditional and too general in scope. The healthcare system in Belgium is also hampered by long waiting lists, full of people 'with a genuine request for support'. Not only are those who miss appointments left to cope on their own, but, when the therapy fails, they are accused of an unwillingness to change ('blaming the victim'). Healthcare services portray these people as hopeless cases, which serves only to confirm their already low self-esteem. Homeless people with mental health issues are often also portrayed as 'care avoiders'.

(free translation) 'Homelessness... people flee in isolation to preserve what remains of their dignity, and this almost checkmates the interventive carers' (Kal, 2001, p. 50).

The word 'almost' in the above quote is vital here. I have heard Dutch colleagues use the term 'careful care seekers' instead of 'worrying care avoiders'. The new term puts the ball in the healthcare professional's court. S/he has to prove her/himself. The healthcare professional must make a sustained effort to reach these people, who have already had so many setbacks in their lives that they may not trust anyone, let alone healthcare professionals. 'Unconditional help' based on presence would appear to offer an answer to the distress. Andries Baart in the words of Doortje Kal again, writes:

> (free translation) '(presence theory) takes the weakest as the measure of quality and if there is nothing more to be achieved, it does not abandon those in need of care', and also: 'good help is recognisable in that it serves the weakest or most problematic help seeker and not the best off or the better or the cleverer'.
>
> (Kal, 2001, p. 50)

It is odd that rough-sleepers in Belgium receive little or no support from mental healthcare services, and that the dynamic of scarcity described above in relation to homeless people in the psychiatric system, is not recognised and acknowledged, so that they are often viewed as resistant to treatment. In this book, we would like to make a case for integrated care for the homeless, no matter where they are staying, be it on the streets, in a halfway house or the psychiatric system. This means listening to their life stories and traumas, and combining this with housing, financial support measures, home counselling... The healthcare professional him/herself can use quartermaking to this effect, to find or create these resources and so, later, detach from the institution.

In the Netherlands in 2000 and 2001 a survey was taken of group leaders in night shelters (Marius Nuy, *De nacht van Nederland*, 2001).

The survey revealed that healthcare professionals at the night shelter saw homelessness as an irreversible situation. This was in reference to their own commitment and the common belief that people would eventually regain a roof over their heads, because, without that belief, no one could do the job. On the other hand, the survey also revealed that healthcare professionals witness homeless people not finding a home and ascribe the reasons for this to them.

It is said that homeless people are not persistent enough, or that it is in their nature not to grapple with the problems (Marius Nuy, *De nacht van Nederland*, 2001, p. 53). I have seen this attitude for myself in practice. Healthcare professionals may believe that they do a good job, but that it is in the nature of the patient to not make use of this help. In my experience, healthcare professionals also appear to blame the failure of their work on the clients themselves. It is this mistrustful attitude on the part of the healthcare professional that makes the client maintain a fearful distance from the professional. The client feels misunderstood.

Healthcare professionals who want to effect real change in the situation of people are often constrained by their organisation and the core tasks associated with institutional functioning. Ultimately, this limitation contributes to the so-called professional distance which healthcare professionals maintain in order to carry out their work (Andries Baart, *Uitwisseling tussen Werner van de Vrede en Andries Baart over Presentiebenadering*, 2020).

What we do on the rehabilitation ward at Sleidinge is take in homeless people with mental ill health. Essentially, we take these people, often without a request for therapeutic help, and help them discover that request, that desire. We try to find out what they find important in live, by listening and by visiting places that are important for them. After many years of psychiatric admissions, previously having been known as 'chronic', people appear to be interested in very little, or experiencing psychosis to the extent that they are unable to give us a clear picture. We start by acknowledging their suffering. The very first thing we do is ignore the notes from previous admissions. Most of the time these just describe the history of the illness, not the person's life. At this new admission, we wish to be someone who gets to know the person behind the patient. It is about belief in the encounter, and about the hope that this can inspire. The process we commence with the help seeker is not a re-run of all the previous techniques and procedures. It is based on a belief in the unique nature of the bond between us, the help provider and the help seeker. We go in search of the flame that burns within. We look for what drives him/her, what touches him/her: that which is deeply buried below homelessness and long stays on psychiatric wards. We do it by walking alongside him/her, often literally. Not always in a group, but mostly individually. A practical issue of any kind, or an expression, of sadness say, or especially anger, can be a sign of that flickering flame. We also accompany these help seekers in their search for a suitable new place to live. Whether living independently, in sheltered housing or with home support, their preference is of paramount importance. For those who do not know which way to go, we begin with stacks of information. We introduce the idea of sheltered accommodation, for example, by inviting people who are already in sheltered housing to the ward. Some of these residents may even become a home buddy. This provides volunteer work for people who already live in sheltered accommodation. The support does not end before a home is found, and, once a home is in place, we consider follow-up home support. If follow-up support is unavailable, because the client is too far down the waiting list, we provide at-home support ourselves. In the case of sheltered accommodation, we ensure a friendly handover to the future home supporters.

There is nothing better than to experience for yourself the thrill of helping someone back into a home and restoring their sense of freedom after many years of psychiatric care. This reaches its height when, hesitantly and inquisitively, they turn the key in their own front door for the first time. And then, when their name goes up by the doorbell…

On our ward, not only do we ensure that patients find a home, but we take care of the home support, in some cases, while they are on the Fact Team waiting list.

Every home is different when you are providing at-home support, and the interior says something about the person who lives there. I get to know the resident a little better just by going in. A book on the table, a CD, a bag of sweets, a can of coke. There's a sense of what the resident was doing, what he or she was up to before I came in. There is a person living here. I am still very deferential on entering a client's home. I am being allowed in. I am entering a place where someone lives. I am a visitor. Obviously, it is better to prevent a person from losing their home in the first place, and I think that this should be a FACT Team's main line of operation. I have been fortunate enough to spend three years (2012–2015) on one of these teams. It is about the treatment and support of clients in their natural environment. When we began providing home support for clients with mental health issues we discovered methods that work well from a technical point of view. … But we were interested in basic 'strength based' attitudes (C. Rapp, *The strengths model: Case management with people suffering severe and persistent mental illness*, 1988) as well the presence theory (Andries Baart, *Theorie van de presentie*, 2001) mentioned earlier, but what I could not find was an understanding of the essence of our work. What is the point of going to a person's home? What does visiting the home mean to these clients? These questions are inseparable from a number of others, such as what 'living at home' can and should involve. What makes a home a home?

I would like, now, to present a picture of living by drawing on the concepts of time and space. If a resident does not feel at home in her/his house, and if there is no familiarity with the things within it, then living itself is highly problematic and care in the home is advisable. This care is especially recommended if the resident is no longer able to formulate a request for support. Home care is also recommended in the case of residents who have no real perspective of time. It is the problematic attitude to home living that should be the determining factor in the provision of home care. My hope for the future is that the very people who find themselves in this situation will be the target group for case managers. The lack of certain individual characteristics is usually not enough to explain the problems that some people with mental illness may experience. Social factors must always be taken into consideration, such as the availability of decent, affordable rental accommodation, better access to social housing and adequate support from family and in their social environment. And yet we would like to make some room here to examine the individual-related problem that causes a person with mental ill health to run into difficulties when living in a house. In Belgium, we hope this answers the concern from social housing, that they are constantly having clients referred to them who are not 'move-in ready'. Our analysis is made from a phenomenological perspective. Through practical examples, consisting mostly of observations and discussions with clients, for which I have informed consent consisting mostly, we summarise ideas and develop theories on how some people with mental health issues relate to living in a house. Specifically, we look at whether there is a link between mental health issues and the difficulty or impossibility of home living. By 'impossibility of home living' we mean several things: loss of privacy caused by rough sleeping in public, loss of social contact and domestic well-being, difficulties with developing personal potential and a loss of dignity. It is quite remarkable to witness, time and again, how a person's behaviour on a ward can differ dramatically from their behaviour at home. We underestimate the power of people.

Joseph is another of the people I meet through my work on the Fact Team. I visit him at home. When coaching him I get to thinking about how objects like tables and chairs are transformed into homeliness. I ring his bell in the foyer. The speaker crackles. I hear no voice, but I know he is listening. I say my name and hear the door buzz beside me. Joseph has used the entry phone to let me in. I climb the stairs to his apartment. He opens the door incredibly slowly, and I wait for the opening to get big enough for me to step inside. He closes it again and slowly turns the lock. I slow down too and avoid sudden movements. I ask if I can take a seat. He nods slowly, and the hint of a smile crosses his lips. I slide the chair from under the table and sit. Now Joseph pulls the other chair out from under the table, slides it back carefully, turns it very slowly through 180 degrees and sits, hands resting on the backrest. This is the first time ever on one of my visits. On the previous three occasions he has stood bolt upright the whole time, arms folded, half a metre from his door.

There is nothing on the table but a calendar, and, on top of that, a letter. This kitchen is a small, bare space. It has a table, the two chairs, one glass and one fork beside the washing-up bowl. There are no pictures on the wall. He has a TV and a DVD player, which he only ever uses to watch this one music DVD. On top of the TV there is a digital clock radio. The reading of the mail is a ritual. I ask if I should open the letter. He nods. The housing agency is offering him a new and longer tenancy. I advise him to show it to his benefits office. He thinks for a long time before deciding on a date. We talk about his home appliances. He tells me that everything is okay now. A new boiler was fitted recently, and a radiator was replaced.

On my first visit he had many questions about the pilot light. When I told him that there was no need for the boiler to be on in summer, he wanted the exact date for when the flame should be off. When I mentioned the seasons he wondered if the season dates would be of any help. Was it okay to turn the pilot light off on the first day of spring, and then on again on the first day of autumn? That led to a conversation about the exact dates on which spring and autumn begin. Between his words there were extremely long pauses. 'It is complicated,' he said, 'Four seasons. In Congo there are only two: dry season and rainy season.' On the first visit I managed to put his mind at ease. The flame could stay on.

Now he is returning to that conversation. He wants to show me that all is okay. He wants me to see the pilot light on the kitchen gas fire. He stands beside me and shows me the best angle to view it. Then he asks me to look at the pilot light in the gas fire upstairs. When I move to follow him upstairs he advises me to bring my satchel with me. I tell him that it is okay to leave it where it is. He checks that the door is locked. Obviously, he thinks my satchel might get stolen.

This is the first time I have been upstairs. It is a fairly big loft and, aside from the heater, it contains a bench and a two-piece cabinet: a base and a top. He asks me to look at the pilot light for this heater. I don't see it immediately, so he slides the grate to the side a little. I feel the heat, but can't see the flame. He gives me directions until finally I see it. Then he slowly and carefully slides back the grate.

He slides the cabinet top to the side slightly and looks at me inquisitively: 'Is this okay?' I tell him that the cabinet is made of two pieces, an upper part and a lower part, and that this makes it easy to transport when you move house.

He tells me that the loft will be for his family if they come to visit. It is the first time he has mentioned them. He has three sisters. He arranges them according to place of residence, Belgium and France, and then relationship status. He doesn't tell me their names. Back downstairs, I jot my next appointment down on the calendar and repeat several more times the date of my return. We get back onto the day and month for the start of the seasons. I have an idea to bring next time a map of Ghent. He smiles when he retrieves the names and numbers from memory and uses them to tell me where he has lived. He loves to give long and detailed descriptions of the places he has lived in, with tram lines and street names. When he is asked where he liked living best, the smile disappears. Joseph seems not to understand the question. When it is time to go I ask him to open the door. He does it as slowly and as carefully as when he let me in.

In his book entitled *Naakt geboren* (1999) Jacques De Visscher describes what homeliness is:

(free translation) We know this house accommodates us because so much of what is found there and is used by us every day guides, confirms and is close to our life, but at the same time connects us with elsewhere, with what happens outside the house in the world around us.

(p. 80)

It is the intimacy of the things that connect us with elsewhere, but also with the past. De Visscher distinguishes between objects and things: (free translation) 'Thus, homeliness presupposes the presence of occupants who relate to things in the appropriate sense, who are close to things through their very use' (p. 80).

When talking about people with psychosis he writes:

In an inauthentic home (...) everything appears to have its place but nothing appears to be organically part of a whole, of a physical life. Individuated, things are barely exposed objects, devoid of any impressionability or concern for the world. They reveal so little of their earthly origin. In objects there is no life, they are dead, autistic. In that sense we cannot talk about the objects in the homely house.

(p. 80)

I am very conscious of the objects in Joseph's apartment. They are what De Visscher would describe as 'objects'. This is mostly because there is a loss of naturalness and spontaneity in the way I have to relate, through him, to the objects in his home. He handles them as if they are brittle and fragile. The door opens so slowly that it makes me feel unsafe, especially when he locks it after me. It feels not like a threshold between inside and out, but a barricade. You can hardly call it a welcome. The chairs are under the table when you enter, so there is no invitation to sit. I have to ask if I can take a seat. By sliding the chair from under the table I turn the object into a thing. The chair and the table are connected. I sit at the table. Joseph appears unable to participate in this connection with things. He will remain on his feet for our first three conversations.

For the fourth conversation, the second chair transforms from an object into a thing. But in a hesitant and exploratory way. Joseph does not seem to understand the way of things. He sits down with me, but differently: chair back facing forward, legs apart, hands on backrest. Perhaps, rather than mirroring me, this different seating posture is designed to establish a safe distance between us. Being seated in exactly the same way may be threatening. But something has actually taken place. We are sitting together at the table. The table connects us to the chairs. Two people are together. The unopened letter is on the table. Now that he too is seated at the table it has become a place where we read the letter together.

And there are other objects too. The furniture feels not human, but museum-like. You can look at the pieces. It is what Joseph asks me to do. He asks me to inspect the pilot lights on the gas heater. The heaters are a matter of concern for Joseph. There is the pilot light, and there is the issue of whether it should be on, when it should be on, and when it should be off. I play my part in objectifying the heater. We inspect it together, as an object with a shape, and, deep at its centre, a content: a flame that stays alight. We inspect the flame together. It is okay. It is lit. We go upstairs to inspect the flame. He and I go and find it there. I wonder if by looking at it together we can transform this object into a thing, something he can use to stay warm in the winter, sitting on a chair. And if the cabinet can become a utilitarian object, and no longer something that consists of two parts.

Joseph has lost the spontaneity and naturalness with which an animal inhabits its den, its shell. An animal does not inhabit its den as much as become its den. It is at one with its shell. A human being turns objects into things, creates the connectedness between things, and, for that reason, things can make space for a social event. Joseph appears to be missing these fundamentals. The house that is no more than a shelter is still threatening, because it is not a home, because it is not inhabited. If things are not linked to each other or the user they exist alone and become a source of anxiety. Their presence, unconnected, is best expressed in Sartre's *Nausea* (1987):

> Things are divorced from their names. They are there, grotesque, headstrong, gigantic and it seems ridiculous to call them seats or say anything at all about them: I am in the midst of things, name-less things. Alone, without words, defenceless, they surround me, are beneath me, behind me, above me. They demand nothing, they don't impose themselves: they are there.
>
> (pp. 148, 174)

Joseph's fear of the objects gives me a place in this home. There is a purpose to my visits. He asks me questions about the objects. By being present I try to give answers, in the hope that my answers lay the groundwork, form a base for him. I realise that my answers can sometimes lead to new questions and new problems for him. I take greater care with my answers. He tells me that he often lies awake at night, thinking. By welcoming me into this house, where no one would otherwise come, as part of this home care service, he is humanised, made more human to himself, and things are made whole. My visit gives rise to the possibility of things making space for a social event. I would say that this is almost the essence of home visits to people with mental ill health: the visit produces an encounter.

> (free translation) One of the properties of a thing is that it synthe-sises, collects, and that it gives a place to an event. Objects cannot

31

do this, in their individuation they remove themselves from the world and from everything that concerns us in our daily lives.

(Visscher, 1999, p. 87)

I should briefly identify another aspect of meeting, in that Joseph says the area upstairs is where he will entertain his family when they visit. This space is the guest room. He feels a part of the world, through his family, in this room. It is a place of expectation, like that felt by a man who is about to be a father and already envisages his future child's room. I bear this in mind for my next visits. Might there be a desire to buy furniture, such as a bed, to have his family over? Will the house be more like a home then? Will the door be more like a threshold across which people can be welcomed, rather than a barricade against the outside? Above all, this room will give me the space to talk more about Joseph's family.

Karel's counselling also seems to suggest that the relationship between guest and host is vital of the process. He is difficult to contact. His parents and grandmother ask for help. I support them. Karel is often away from home, which makes his grandmother uneasy. He rides off on his moped. Karel hears voices. He is insulted and harassed by them. This is particularly bad when he takes drugs and stays up all night. On these occasions he is so angered and frustrated by the voices that he throws cups and saucers through the window and smashes up his room. Sometimes he goes out and rips wing mirrors from cars. Beyond supporting his family I think it is important to talk to Karel himself. I call on him regularly, and he only answers the door one in three. Sitting in the living room with him feels very awkward. He says very little, unless he is talking about his voices.

I think it might be easier to connect if we find something enjoyable to do in his home. I suggest making croque-monsieurs. Karel likes the idea. I buy bread, cheese and ham and come over at the arranged time. He doesn't answer the door. Later he will say that he saw me riding off and felt sorry for me after I had gone to all that trouble.

After a new crisis he is involuntarily detained. I now visit the ward with frequent regularity. He can't leave me standing at the door now that he has been admitted. We play billiards on the ward, wander around the neighbourhood, go to the cafeteria. I ride home with him to get his clothes and stay in touch with his grandmother all the while. The team consults regularly. He and I attend the team meetings. Now and again Karel absconds by climbing over the garden wall, and when he does, he uses drugs. On these occasions he is returned by the police or comes back to the institution later. It is still difficult to talk about the things on his mind. Once, when I go round, Karel asks me to come shopping with him. He tells me that the place would feel homelier if there was food in the fridge. He adds that he can't get by on the money he gets. He buys drugs. He asks if I can work out a budget to cover his groceries and no more. This seems like a good idea to me. I have a feeling that it might be a breakthrough. I call his budget manager and ask her to transfer money to the local psychiatric institute every week, so that I can collect it for him and go shopping with him at the same time every Wednesday. I suspect the time has come for me to develop my idea on friendliness. I suggest that we cook when we get home on shopping day.

When we return to his apartment for the first time after shopping, I ask him if he would rather peel the potatoes or wash the vegetables. He says it would be better if I sit at the table while he prepares the food in the kitchen. For me, as a health professional, it feels odd to do nothing. He seems to notice this and gives me some magazines to read. We get into a way of talking that seems to suit him. He disappears into the kitchen, re-emerges for a quick chat while the potatoes boil and then goes back into the kitchen. In the meantime, I work on a few files on my computer. Karel is busy, and I am busy, only on different things. Here and there, between our chores, we talk a little. It seems to work. He is not stressed by the silences that occasionally creep in when we are talking face-to-face. The conversation takes place between flurries of activity; activities that will eventually bring us together to eat. I see now that he was aware of the uneasiness I had felt in our earlier contact. If it happens again he simply disappears into the kitchen, where there are things to be done anyway. He sets the table, and we eat. We do it every Wednesday from then on.

Karel shows me in any case that living it isn't really about friendliness, but the relationship between the host and the guest. He is the host, and I am the person he welcomes in, and that is how he gets to inhabit his apartment. When I see him next week he tells me he cooked for himself on Saturday. It is through my presence, my visits, that this apartment becomes a place that he inhabits. It is by looking after someone else that he rediscovers the ability to look after himself. 'Odd, though,' he says. 'I cooked every day on the psychiatric ward. But back home, I stopped.' There was no one else to cook for at the time.

Going into the home really does do something for the people you visit, provided the relationship is always one of host and guest.

2.2 The Experience of Time

The emotional biography of our childhood homes goes beyond the architectural envelopes they provide for our mentalized and un-mentalized erotic, hostile, tender, civic, and spiritual aspirations. Internalized, their corridors, closets, and cloisters function as life-long psychic retreats and springboards for mental rejuvenation Driven by naive hope, we visit them in actuality and come back wounded. But then the plump nursemaid of nostalgia leads us back to those very streets and lampposts and we return with a poem in our hands. As we grow old, life's intoxication gradually changes into tipsy indifference, but arriving at our eternal resting place we are unexpectedly clear-eyed. We see that we have ended up where we started from. Our childhood homes might have been lost but childhood itself has turned out to be our home. Loyally and forever.
(Salman Akhtar, *The Homes of Childhood: Spaces of Love, Dread, and Play*, Analytical Spaces Workshop, London, 14 July 2012)

Contact with Leo teaches me a lot about time and the dilapidation of the home. Leo is involuntarily detained. His neighbours have complained about how his dilapidated house is damaging theirs. On entering Leo's home the police make a grim discovery: mould and dry rot everywhere... The house is uninhabitable. Leo stopped paying the water and electricity bills a long time ago, and has been cut off. With no water to flush the toilet, he has been using the cellar. Letters and documents delivered by the postman over the years have all been kept and neatly stacked unopened. After a short stay on the locked ward Leo is transferred to the rehabilitation ward. The team have tried to make him see that his house is in need of repair. But it hasn't worked, and an administrator has been appointed. The house is fit only for demolition. Leo refuses to live anywhere else, sheltered accommodation included. Nothing can be better than his own property, the place where he felt at home. He is very angry at what the neighbours have done to him and brings it up in discussion every day, his only request being that he return to his house immediately. Leo gets so distraught at our reply that we begin to fear a suicide attempt. After much discussion, involving no more at first than listening to his request for discharge, we discover more about what makes Leo tick. His neighbour, a policeman, threatened him with his weapon. Leo felt that the man was using all kinds of strange powers in an attempt to influence him. He said he knew of his neighbour's plans to murder him. The disconnection of the water and electricity was also perceived as a hostile move by the neighbour. And so Leo became more and more insular. He denies that his house is dilapidated and says there is nothing wrong with it: it hasn't been tampered with over the years and he has kept it in its original condition. He has kept everything delivered by the postman, even the bills. He threw nothing away. All is fine, as long as you save everything.

When things wear alongside us, this is a hallmark of intimacy with things, or so De Visscher argues (1999).

In his book *Sculpting in Time* the director Tarkovski refers to the Japanese concept of 'saba'.

In his account of Japan the journalist Ovchinnikov wrote:

> It is considered that time, per se, helps to make known the essence of things. The Japanese therefore see a particular charm in the evidence of old age. They are attracted to the darkened tone of an old tree, the ruggedness of a stone, or even the scruffy look of a picture whose edges have been handled by a great many people. To all these signs of age they give the name, saba, which literally means "rust".
>
> (Tarkovsky, 1989, p. 30)

It is this residue, this patina, this rust, that the Japanese refer to as 'saba'. The wear is what gives things their familiarity. It harks back to an earlier time.

But signs of wear can also be paired with getting tired of things, with a quest for change, the desire to repair things, move house or seek renewal. More than that, where living is concerned this becomes necessary in the end.

In her essay 'Thuis: een plaats om beu te worden' (1997) (free translation) 'Home: A Place to Tire of', Patricia De Martelaere goes in search of what living means to each of us. You maintain your house, work on it, enjoy the open fire in the winter, the balcony in the summer. You move around the house unselfconsciously. This helps you save energy for other activities, but in the process the house becomes a daily grind. You tire of the house and fight this in all kinds of ways. You can either move to a new house, or, if that's too expensive, move within the house: refurbish the rooms or use them for another purpose. You introduce novelty in an attempt to escape the grind. Newness brings beauty. De Martelaere (1997, pp. 10–12) writes that this is because living has an irrevocable ugliness. After a while, even the finest interior generates feelings of oppression, resentment and loathing when inhabited day in, day out, year in, year out by the same people, using the same old body language. One way to escape this is to invite friends, neighbours or guests in. From them it will be easy to elicit the sigh of amazement that decayed, long ago, into a sigh a weariness on the dweller's part. This analysis shows that living involves a dynamic that each of us has trouble with:

> (free translation) The real art of living is the art of moving home. He who moves home loses everything, starts again as a child. (...) Moving home goes with disorganisation and disarray, but also with thrill and passion. Everything is seen again for the first time.
>
> (De Martelaere, 1997, p. 11)

Advertisers present living as if it were all about building a nest where you can be safe and secure around the hearth in the winter and on the terrace in the summer. The reality is very different. A house wears out, falls apart, slips into disrepair. The house, originally conceived to protect people, soon becomes a place for people to protect. The dream becomes a chore; if the work is not done, it collapses.

Leo appears to champion the immutability of his home at all costs. It is as if he possesses the never-changing dream home, where there is no such thing as the daily grind, and the protection afforded by the walls actually does keep a hostile world at bay. Once built, the nest is complete for all time. There is no need to move house, inside or outside.

Leo does not notice that time has passed, and that time itself has changed his house. In his timeless state, dilapidation does not register. Given that he associates change with hostility, he clings ever more stubbornly to the ideal of a safe nest, unchangeable, in a changing world.

If objects become things, then familiarity with them exists, and things become a place for an event which is social by definition. It seems to me, when we think about living, that besides familiarity there is also the important notion of time, which relates not only to 'saba' but to degradation, renewal, moving house... This notion of time also relates to historicisation, to an existence in which present and future take their meaning from the past, but a past that is also reshapeable by present events. In other words, living is not just a sense of well-being in the home, a feel of home. It comes with the acknowledgement that living is a task, a job, in the sense that a home has to be worked on, to be maintained, and, if it is not, the place we inhabit is vulnerable to neglect, even decay.

Some people have a strange perception of time, through which they do not experience dilapidation for what it is. With other people, there is a clear link between dilapidation and early traumatic experiences. The key thing here is the childhood home. This path will eventually allow us to take a closer look at the relationship between living and language.

Dilapidation is a clear sign that something has gone wrong with a person's stay in their house. Neglect of the home does not always indicate the same issues. The first big question relates to how the client perceives dilapidation. This is the basis for deciding the rest of the treatment. Is the resident (still) aware of the dilapidation, and can the subject be raised with him/her? If not, is his/her refusal to talk based on shame? And, if s/he is unaware of the dilapidation, is it because dilapidation means something else to him/her? Does s/he understand what dilapidation is?

> Johan shows me the crack in the ceiling plaster. He looks at me again: 'It's the neighbours'. He nods. He doesn't know who they are, but they are there. They have done this. They must have a house

key, because they have been in, he adds. He points to the fire extinguisher on the landing and says that it is not on its bracket, but on the ground. 'Look!' He shows me the cracks in the hallway. And that door downstairs is always open. People forget to close it, or leave it open deliberately. The more he points out, the angrier he gets. Signals. I have to believe him.

Jacques has mice. He hears voices, and they send him messages through the mice. Jacques watches how the mice behave, because he wants to follow the messages. There is nothing else he can do. He wants to know what is going to happen around him, and happen to him.

The clients in the examples above seem to have no concept of dilapidation, or at least they do not think of it as many of us do. The basic principle that things change with time, or, more particularly, that things fall into disrepair as time passes, appears not to have registered. For some, dilapidation may even have taken on a meaning that does not coincide with the passage of time. Dilapidation has meaning in relationship terms. In which case, matter is no longer dispassionate towards the person who inhabits it. Deterioration is not a law of physics, but intentional, purposeful, and the residents are passive at its centre. They suffer, and sense a loss of control. It leaves them as a fascinated, spellbound victim. It eats up all of their attention and leads to apathy. The changing of matter signals something else, something beyond their influence that relates to them, the inhabitants. When mice and rats suddenly appear in his home, Jacques does not take it as a sign of dilapidation, but a sign from God. He sees them as signals from another world, and they are often very threatening. It alarms him. The fear, powerlessness and apathy can give rise to anger and aggression. Being at the mercy of something that changes and works as a signal is very far removed from seeing natural change and deterioration, against which action has to be taken, in the form of repairs.

In Belgium, requests for support rarely come in from these clients, given their concept of dilapidation. As a healthcare professional you try to develop a bond that enables you to get permission to act against the dilapidation. It is important to understand the client's view of his/her environment, and his/her explanation and interpretation of this environment. It is obvious that this interpretation can be very individual and surprising, but the insight can help you understand the client's experience of the environment and perhaps find a way, based on that interpretation, to be certain that the client eventually has the repairs done and allows cleaners in to keep the home clean and tidy. And all before it is too late, before the landlord decides to evict, before the home is utterly destroyed and there is nothing else for it but a long stay on a psychiatric ward.

For a number of other clients, their issues in their homes relate more or less directly to the past.

> Take Jan, for example. He is unable to stay inside his home. He spends the night in the woods or the fields. As a child Jan would be hauled from his bed by his mother, along with his brothers and sisters, when his father came home drunk. There would always be an enormous scene, in which their mother would be so severely battered that the children frequently feared for her life. The father would sometimes threaten to shoot her. In that case, their mother would gather up the children and flee from the house in the middle of the night, and the family would be taken in by the neighbours, in a strange house. For Jan as a boy the strange house signified safety, whereas the parental home was associated with hostility. After a row his mother would always return, when asked by her now sober husband, and bring her children back to the place where life, especially sleep, was unsafe. Now, more than thirty years later, Jan can only stay in one place for a few months, and he often sleeps rough for a few nights at a time. He sleeps in woods, garages, empty buildings... He often sleeps rough after a row or a difference of opinion. It seems that he feels safer outside, in the unknown, than inside. After a few days, sometimes weeks, he returns to the psychiatric ward in a state of self-neglect.

Traumatic childhood experiences play a big part in the way people live, especially if the traumas were experienced in the family home, when the child was at a very tender age. Gaston Bachelard (*Poetics of space*, 1969, p. 14) talks about old abodes, the houses we used to live in and the memories we have of those places. He claims that previous homes are indelibly written into us, and not just as memories. He writes that we cannot know ourselves in time without the concept of space. We are incapable of reliving a period of time without reference to space. But our memories actually store an entire spatial experience of time. Thus a person collects all kinds of spaces over a lifetime, filled with memories, compressed time.

Then there are daydreams. Bachelard links the earliest childhood daydreams in the childhood home to home living. The images carried within us, and accumulated by daydreaming in our childhood home, are in compressed time and so their progression is compressed. This is because the daydream contains a clear, active component. It is processed as a narrative (*Poetics of space*, 1964, p. 15).

Daydreaming in the home, the child has a sense of well-being. Bachelard says that this kind of dreaming is not the same as fantasising, or, for that matter, creating fantastical, previously unseen forms from nothing. Imagination largely involves the transformation of images and is virtually synonymous with metamorphosis (*Poetics of space*, 1969, p. 17).

Childhood daydreaming in the home, associated with a sense of well-being at home, tends to be more unconscious and so fundamental that it precedes recollection or memory. This is why, when seeking to return to the fundaments of our well-being, we are not historians but poets. The daydreams that coincide with living may be the very things that conjure up a space for us to store the memories in. Thus, the imagery of the house works in two directions: the images are as much in us as we are in them. We 'house' not only our memories, but the things we have forgotten: 'our soul' is a dwelling place. And because we remember our 'houses' and 'rooms', we learn to 'dwell' in ourselves. We comfort ourselves by reliving memories of protection. Our memories of the outside world will never have the same tone as memories of home, and by recollecting them we add material to our dreams. We associate home with safety, warmth and love.

In *Hold Still*, photographer Sally Mann discusses the Welsh word 'hiraeth', which refers to the pain of longing for lost places from the past. She talks about place pain:

> It always refers to a near umbilical attachment to a place, not just free-floating nostalgia or a droopy houndlike wistfulness or the longing we associate with romantic love. No, this is a word about the pain of loving a place.

(2015, p. 175)

You may wonder what it is about our former dwelling places that remains present in us if trauma is the main thing we associate with them. From the earliest times in life, living can be a cause for disquiet and insecurity. A cause for suffering which cannot be described in words, because the experiences are so intensely and profoundly traumatising that they cannot be named, and because they occur at so tender an age that the child is unable to recognise their experience as abnormal. Now and then, fortunately, when the child suffers these traumas, there is a silent witness, a friend or relative who is able to put the abnormality of the situation into words without necessarily intervening. He or she will arrange for a holiday somewhere else, for example, to allow something of the child's suffering to be voiced and represented. This representation is what the child may later return to in healing discussions with the healthcare professional.

> Lucia is admitted to the ward. She is keen to tell any willing or unwilling listener about her knowledge of sewing and knitting and other creative hobbies. Those who are not interested, or contradict her, are either too idle to learn something new or envious of her

knowledge. She feels misunderstood and lives in a world of idiots and know-it-alls. People who chat about the weather or never rise above small talk are a waste of time. They don't realise how important real knowledge is. Lucia is not all that popular with the others. And she seems aware of it. She says she is so smart that she can't find anyone who can talk to her. Her reassuring explanation for her lack of friends and acquaintances is: 'I am too smart, and that is why I am alone'. Her loneliness is a misfortune, and one which she can proudly bemoan, for it is the result of an achievement. This step takes Lucia from a passive position to an active one, and gives her greater comfort. Lucia visits often, and when she comes she does all the talking. She sees me as someone who listens to her knowledge... She tells me what she has read in the magazines she buys. She leaves with a sense of satisfaction.

It takes quite some time before Lucia opens up about her past and her sadness. She was a terrible pupil it seems, because she wasn't interested in school. The others thought she was stupid and bullied her. Defending herself only got her into trouble with the teachers. She was relatively old when she stopped wetting the bed. Lucia tells me that she is lonely and invites me to visit. In her house, time appears to have stopped: the wardrobe in her parents' bedroom contains the clothes of her long-dead mother, and on the mantlepiece stands the figure of Mary to which the family prayed to save her terminally-ill sister. Lucia talks about her past in reference to the things in her house. But not for too long, for fear of making her nightmares worse. It was bad in the past, and she would rather blot it out. She was stupid then, and she wants to catch up on her knowledge through study. Her knowledge of the past has to be covered by a knowledge of creative pursuits. Lucia attempts to make changes in the house. A new bathroom, when she meets a man who would like to live with her, a kitchen extension: she does it all alone. But she always abandons the building work before it is finished. She knows the importance of looking after things and turns to her family for help: the laundry, the cleaning, the gardening... She doesn't think she gets enough help. We suggest a home help service to take care of the practical things. Lucia wants her family's opinion on this. The family, especially her eldest sister, rejects everything we propose on the subject. She doesn't want strangers in the house. But she herself is too busy to come around more often. The sister also has the feeling of being all alone.

We want to know what is going on here, and invite the family over. We view them as partners in this task. The two sisters accept our invitation. The eldest speaks at length about their traumatic childhood experiences. Lucia probably knows what will be said and chooses not to attend. The information surprises us. We could never have known just how bad it was for them. The mother died when Lucia is young, a significant event in her life. A helpless but dictatorial father took over the housekeeping, with Lucia's elder sister who was still a child herself. The sisters tell us that life became a living hell after their mother's death. The eldest sister did her absolute best to take care of the family. But she was far too young for the task. Her father and aunts were more obstructive than anything else. She did everything she could to present a picture to the outside world. But Lucia got hardly any attention, stayed with acquaintances for a while and was only ever included by the sisters if there were battles to be fought when they were deprived or disadvantaged. With time the family members married and flew the nest, and the father went into a care home. The father died and left the parental home to Lucia. For years now she has lived there on her own.

The eldest sister feels responsible for Lucia, but, more than that, she feels guilty for her inability to take over after her mother's death. She recognises that by continuing to help Lucia she is endangering her own health as well as her relations with her own family. She still sees herself as the head of the original family and tries, to no avail, to enlist other members of the family to help Lucia. A few lend a hand, reluctantly, but only then through a sense of loyalty to the elder sister. They don't want outsiders or busybodies in. Just relatives. They have a terrible sense of shame. The shame that others may sense the trauma when they enter this house, is too great to allow strangers in. It turns out that it is extremely hard for most family members, and the eldest sister in particular, to enter the house, which has been the scene of so many terrible events. There is a sense of physical revulsion to be overcome.

A few months later, the two sisters ask to see us again. They talk at length about their huge concerns for Lucia, but mostly about their feelings of guilt towards her. The loyalty that holds the traumatised members of this family together, and rests on shame and hiding the truth from the outside world, seems to present a serious obstacle. This is how things have been in Lucia's family for years. Helping the family process the shame and guilt opens the possibility for the eldest sister to give more time to her new family, her husband and children, and to allow 'strangers', a cleaning service, to enter the parental home in which Lucia still lives.

Lucia suffered a great deal through the dictatorial behaviour of her deeply grieving father. She wants to stay in the family home, with all its secrets, at all costs, because it was left to her by her father. For Lucia, moving home would mean turning her back on the only positive contact she has ever had with her father, this gift.

41

But, then again, staying means being forever faced with traumas she would sooner forget. The only option is to talk about what happened. Only then will it be possible to see through the terrible events and identify the father as a man who was incapable of raising his children after the death of his wife. Lucia is still a long way from reaching this realisation.

I tell Lucia about the conversation with her sisters. It should also give her room to change. I tell her that they find it extremely difficult to enter the house she lives in. Lucia is reluctant, and even misses the odd appointment, which has never happened before, but she puts her talk of creativity aside for a while and tells me the story of her mother, and that of her father, whom, unlike her sisters, she never forsakes. She was proud to be given the house by her father.

It would seem that the initial steps have been taken. It is to be hoped that Lucia understands the message that the family secrets are open to discussion. Periods of inpatient care, outpatient care and full discharge follow in quick succession, but there seems to have been a shift. During the admission Lucia picks up, feeling somewhere between excited and euphoric. Her physical complaints are now invariably associated with the house she lives in: a leaky stove, the cold, the radiation from the TV screen, the toxic plants in the garden. She tells us that she is allergic to them. The house she inhabits appears to be poisoning her. Is she beginning to see that the house, left to her by her father, is a poison chalice? Will she, like her sisters before her, leave the scene of her past behind her? Occasionally she even talks about moving house, to sheltered accommodation, to which she was vehemently opposed before.

The traumatic events leave an image that cannot be processed through recollection, that cannot be reshaped and cannot be affected by the function of forgetting. Is it possible that these images have become frozen precisely because no narrative has been supplied through daydreams? The act of processing events through daydreams and associating safety and security with the place of those daydreams, is unfulfilled.

In the case of daydreaming, the subject takes an active stance, whereas in the case of trauma, suffering prevails. No stance is taken, but passivity comes in. No space can be established in which to stay. Where space cannot be created to hold compressed time, the subject can only ever attempt to wriggle free of the passivity retrospectively. It is not done by remembering, by processing this image, but by reliving the trauma. It is remarkable how the passive attitude to living comes across as problematic in our very first case studies. Lucia is engulfed by nightmares, through which she relives the traumatic events of the past. She also relives them by looking repeatedly at the most horrific images of the Holocaust, and taking pride in having the boldness to look at them. The powerlessness and shame she feels about the horror of her own past are papered over by the pride and power with which she is able to withstand a more universal horror, that of the Second World War. You might say that the pride with which she displays her knowledge of the concentration camps is proportional to her shame over the personal horror she endured. It is too painful to acknowledge the sheer powerlessness of the past, to view herself as a victim. Lucia seems to accuse herself of stupidity because of her disinterest at school. The mechanisms she uses to keep the pain of these memories at bay, such as forcing herself to look at images of the Holocaust, reveal what she seeks to achieve: mastery over this horrific past. However, by choosing to look at the wartime images, an active stance, Lucia runs through the horrors again, without processing them.

The alterations she would like to make in the home can be interpreted in the same way. Lucia attempts to change the dreaded backdrop of her traumatic past in the hope of undoing the trauma in the process. She wants a new kitchen but stops the work before it is completed. She wants to make the home a safer place. She would like to turn it into a cosy nest, fit for her to live in, but she is unsuccessful. The construction work, once started, remains unfinished. The new ruins are witnesses, monuments, to her failed attempts to create something from a material that refuses to be processed in this way. Lucia tries to alter the space itself to process the memories, to undo them in her mind. But, given the trauma, she has no safety-related daydream memories on which to build. Remodelling the home to bring about mental change is no better than cutting a person from a photograph to change your memories of an event. The jagged edge left by the scissors is a permanent reminder of the unendurable pain.

The more I come to know Lucia the more respect I have for her and her ability to bounce back. I listen more attentively and intensively when she comes to visit and shows me her knowledge. I tell her how strong and smart I think she is and how wonderful it is that she has an interest in all these things.

Could the scene of Lucia's childhood home be brought into a therapeutic session? Would she be able to dig up old memories through objects? Speaking about these objects may very well create a new dynamic. Perhaps the congealed image can produce a narrative. But it seems difficult here to combine the home as a place for therapy with the home as a place to live. The objects may help when it comes to talking, but if talking elicits too many nightmares, it must be possible to leave these things as they are and move away from them. In time, the house will cease to function as a home.

In his text *Het (foto)archief* (The photo archive), Dirk Lauwaert describes how children empty the parental home after their parents' death. How they go from one room to another choosing things, and then, afterwards, there are things that nobody wants: (free translation) 'What they want and don't want, is what they want and don't want to remember' (Lauwaert, 2011).

When things are removed from the parental home they take on a new significance. The parents lived among them, and the children who choose them, take them away, have decided to live with them. A move which Lucia is unable to make. She is still living among the things. These things cannot take on a new significance. It might be necessary for her to leave the home. The fact that she is beginning to talk about sheltered accommodation is a good sign.

In Paul Auster's novel *Moon Palace* (1989), the main character is an illegitimate child, 11 years old when he loses his mother. He goes to live with his only relative: uncle Victor. They get along really well and it is a difficult moment when uncle Victor, a clarinettist, goes on tour with his group 'The Moon Men', leaving the 18-year-old lead character behind.

He lives in New York, in a studio apartment on the fifth floor. He is scared in the dark, shadowy room until, on the second or third evening of his stay there, he looks out and spies, between two buildings, a neon advertising sign with the words 'Moon Palace'. It is the advertising board for a Chinese restaurant. The words are like a message to him, because they refer to his uncle Victor's band, and he misses his uncle very much. On seeing the neon lights his fears disappear, and the room he inhabits seems to become a place with internal meaning. He suddenly realises that he is in the right place, and that he was predestined to live in the little apartment.

The right words can give you a feeling of home. Not the words 'done roaming' or 'home sweet home' on the front door of a house but words that actually signify something individual. There was once a client who emphasised her maternal role very strongly and would only stay in one wing of our clinic, the 'Mater Dei'. There is no greater mother than the mother of God, of course.

To feel happy in one's home, it is not enough to be materially well off. Feeling at home is more than being somewhere comfortable, where it is warm in the winter, cool in the summer and dry when it rains. People can cope with, even survive, a shortfall. It is a dangerous illusion to think that we can make it up. In this sense Hubert Van Hoorde in *Psychiatrie en psychoananalyse* (2010) writes: (free translation) 'The home was first sought as accumulated emptiness, as a shrine to the lost object, that cannot be found in the realities'.

This lost object is the unattainable object of our desires. It is language itself that has created the shortfall, and so it will be in the language that we are able to live. For, if nostalgia transports us back to the old avenue and parks where we once lived, we will invent a poetic phrase to remember it, such as invented by W. De Rijck 'Here Lives My House' (Hartmann en Draaisma, *Hier woont mijn huis/here lives my home*, 2012), and in that sense the living is done in the words. It is living in language.

It seems that language is our earliest abode. It originated in the childhood home. The many rooms and corridors in which we played formed spaces in our mind, which are greater than the actual rooms we knew. When we visit them after years of being away we are disappointed. It is only through language, not a story but a poem, that we rediscover part of those original spaces. At the end of our life, we notice that our childhood houses have gone, but that our childhood itself has become our home. It is not like this for everyone. When a childhood was so problematic that the blissful day-dreams associated with living become nightmares, living at home cannot be taken for granted. And even in the case of those who are 'furthest away', where living in a house is concerned, we find a certain logic. It is a very personal logic, which often relates to fear and desperation, brought about by delusions and hallucinations. It is important for us as healthcare professionals to try to share our clients' fear and desperation at living at home, to learn how to unravel that logic and develop a grasp of it. Only when this process has begun can a bond be forged between the healthcare professional and the client, and can the client open up to the healthcare professional. At that point, the healthcare professional becomes an essential mediator between the client and the social housing service. This is what allows him/her to put the patient at ease on the subject of 'move-in readiness' and to offer a response to the difficulties that can sometimes affect a person's living at home.

References

Salman Akhtar, The homes of childhood: Spaces of love, dread, and play. Analytical Spaces Workshop, London, 14 July 2012.

Paul Auster, *Moon palace*, London, Faber & Faber, 1989.

Andries Baart, *Een theorie van de presentie*, Utrecht, Uitgeverij Lemma B.V., 2001.

Andries Baart, Uitwisseling tussen Werner van de Vrede en Andries Baart over Presentiebenadering Present. *Vakblad Sociaal Werk*, 21, 21–23, 2020.

Gaston Bachelard, *The poetics of space*, Boston, MA, Beacon Press, 1969.

Lilanthi Balasuriya, Eliza Buelt and Jack Tsai, The never-ending loop: Homelessness, psychiatric disorder, and mortality. *Psychiatric Times*, 37(5), 12–14, 2020.

Sanne Bloemink, Traumaparadox. *De Groene Amsterdammer*, no. 9, 2016.

Koning Boudewijnstichting, Dak en thuisloosheid tellen om de problematiek beter aan te pakken, persbericht, 2022, https://www.kbs-frb.be/nl/dak-en-thuisloosheid-tellen-om-de-problematiek-beter-aan-te-pakken.

S. Mann, Hold Still, a memoir with photographs, Boston, Little, Brown and Company, 2015.

P. De Martelaere, Thuis, een plaats om beu te worden. In *Verrassingen essays*, Amsterdam, J.M.Meulenhoff bv., pp.7–21, 1997.

J. De Visscher, *Naakt geboren, over herbergzaamheid, lijfelijkheid, subjectiviteit en wereldlijkheid*, Leende, Damon, 1999.

E. Hartmann and D. Draaisma, *Hier woont mijn huis/here lives my home*, Lannoo, Tielt, 2012.

Doortje Kal, *Kwartiermaken. Werken aan ruimte voor mensen met een psychiatrische achtergrond*, Amsterdam, Boom, 2001.

Dirk Lauwaert, Het fotoarchief. In *De witte raaf*, Brussels, edition 149, January–February 2011, p. 1.

Sendhil Mulainathan and Eldar Shafir, *Scarcity. Why having too little means so much*, New York, Times Books, 2013.

C. Rapp, *The strengths model: Case management with people suffering severe and persistent mental illness*, New York, Oxford Press, 1988.

J.-P. Sartre, *Nausea*, Amsterdam, Arbeiderspers, 1987.

Hubert Van Hoorde, Psychoanalyse, lijfelijkheid en wonen. *De Uil van Minerva*, 4(3). doi: https://doi.org/10.21825/uvm.v4i3.1243, 1988.

Tarkovsky A. *Sculpting in time: Reflections on the cinema*, Austin, University of Texas Press, p. 30, 1989.

3

CARE IN THE COMMUNITY
Recovery

3.1 Introduction: A Practical Example of Recovery and Quartermaking

The following account of my experience coaching a couple is from my time on the FACT Team. It offers a chance to discuss the differences between recovery and quartermaking, as well as the points of overlap.

> John and Clara, partners, are referred to our team by the probation service. In repeated efforts to resolve the couple's problems the probation officer has been in touch with several support organisations and psychiatric units. Things can get pretty stormy, even violent, when the couple argue. They tend to binge drink. To diffuse the situation one of them, usually the man, is often detained. An attempt has been made to separate them, or at least persuade them to spend more time apart. There is a theory among the healthcare professionals that the man and woman spend too much time under each other's feet, hence all the stress. For our initial meeting we decide to invite them to the office. We are a little fearful, given the reports of aggressive behaviour. Safety is uppermost in our minds. The woman tells us that her children have given up on her. The man tries to help by taking her side against the children. He sees this as supporting her. The woman says she would prefer it if he did nothing, because all that happens when he takes sides is that her relationships with the children get worse. We manage to convey to him that the woman would prefer him to listen, to help take the strain, but to do nothing. He finds this extremely difficult. He doesn't like to see her suffering. His first instinct is to make something happen, to do something, to stop all the hurt.
>
> We reassure them that we see them as a couple, as two people who love each other dearly. And that for us, as well as them, it is about being able to show their love for each other in a way that suits

DOI: 10.4324/9781003220015-4

them both. This picture puts their minds at rest. The couple are assigned a case manager.

The first crisis occurs. The woman is on the phone in tears. We attend and discover that there is nothing we can actually do. They argue in front of us, as if we're not there. When we phone the next day, concerned, the problem seems to have blown over, and they make light of it without actually denying it. We decide to set the visiting frequency ourselves; once a week, and, for the sake of convenience, at the same time every Wednesday. The woman talks about her past, her parents, her traumatic childhood. We touch on her low self-esteem and her difficult relationships with her children. It involves listening a lot, or being present, and just the very occasional interpretation.

In an evaluation session, after eighteen months of coaching, the team wonders if there is any real point to what we are doing. We visit regularly, and little appears to be changing. The crises keep coming, and so do the complaints. We have given up on the idea of having either admitted to the ward when tensions run high or complaints escalate. It simply doesn't work. The team members' opinions differ on whether we are having an effect, so we decide to ask the couple themselves. The answer takes us somewhat by surprise. They both report a noticeable improvement in their quality of life since we started visiting. For the first time in a long while they feel that people in general, and healthcare professionals in particular, see them as people. With us they don't feel like patients. We haven't made an issue of their drinking, and we are willing to address the things that they find important. They truly appreciate our listening to their life stories as well as offering help with the paperwork, finances and social housing agency. The house is frequently in need of repair, which can be a long time coming. Our help has prompted the housing agency to get their technical staff on the job right away. In other words, we see two very happy people, and their happiness spurs us on.

On a Monday morning I run through my diary and notice a conflict with our Wednesday appointment. Something has come up unexpectedly. I call the woman and ask if I can come today, a few days earlier than planned. She says that she would prefer me not to. She tells me that she looks terrible as she is still getting over a heavy drinking session at the weekend. A while ago, they stopped drinking on Sundays, she tells me, to clear their heads before I come over on Wednesday. They find the visit so important that they want to enjoy it to the full, or be sober in other words. Unbeknown to us, the visits have affected their drinking habits, or at least their drinking pattern. They have something other than alcohol to look forward to. Something worthwhile: so worthwhile that they want to experience it sober. It is an evolutionary trend that will continue. We observe a gradual reduction in their alcohol consumption and a lower incidence of conflict between them.

This is the recovery aspect. We do not focus on crises or problems, but on the person, and this attitude will lead to fewer crises in the end. Two important pillars of the work are being present and listening to a person's life story. Our getting to grips with very specific requests for support, such as filling out forms and complaining to the landlord when the heating system breaks, makes them feel that there are people out there who believe that they are worth the effort. Now that others consider them worthwhile, they will see themselves as worthwhile too. When saddled with problems people often lack the courage or energy to do something like write a letter of complaint. Pitching in to write the letter and, in doing so, improving a person's living circumstances, can help them find the energy and courage to live. With a little practical help, away from all the other problems, they can devote more bandwidth to longer-term thinking, and this frees up the energy needed to tackle the drinking problem, which you, the healthcare professional, do not need to focus on directly. To labour the point about the negative effects of alcohol, or press for an admission to rehab, is to re-stigmatise them and narrow their identity to 'addict', which is dehumanising.

Quite a few of the healthcare professionals before us have correctly identified the couple's isolation. They are ashamed of themselves, each other and their partnership. This doubling or tripling of shame makes them hardly dare show themselves in public. The mirror image that each sees reflected in their partner creates even lower self-esteem, even aggression. We despise in others what we cannot tolerate in ourselves.

The woman seems interested in doing more outside the home. I tell her about the organisations in the community. Organisations I have come to know through my many contacts in the area. I get in touch with a local service centre on her behalf. She hopes to do some sewing and alterations. She used to enjoy this, and her mother was a seamstress. At the introductory meeting we learn that there is a vacancy for a librarian. That sounds fine, she says. She goes once, but not a second time. I don't push it. I notice that she has put going out on the back burner. When, after a while, the local service centre calls and asks if she is planning to return, she is delighted that they have thought about her and haven't forgotten her. She doesn't go back, and then, after an even longer spell, she doesn't dare to. She is ashamed at having stayed away so long. I tell her about a neighbourhood centre in the same area, where you can do sewing. I tell her I am good friends with someone who works there, Nancy, and I talk about how friendly and socially engaged this lady is. We arrange a visit and I bring my client and her husband with me. We are welcomed with open arms. Nancy takes plenty of time to chat with us and the woman in my care is thrilled with the outing. She seems interested and comes twice more before stopping.

Again, we don't make an issue of it. It is a habit of mine to tell my clients about the places I visit and everything they do or provide there. It tells them something about me, the things I do and the people I meet in their community. It also allows me to bring a balanced, positive view of the world to people who are already quite familiar with exclusion. As well as talking about client discrimination and stigmatisation, which I witness at first hand in my work, and about the action we take to counter it, I tell my clients about the very welcoming places where people with fine ideals live and work. At one point I tell my client about a new initiative in the neighbourhood centre: the free box. You bring stuff to put in the box and people take what they want. No need to pay or leave anything in exchange. My client enthuses about this and says that she has lots of second-hand clothes, all branded, from her days as a business manager. She tells me she will pack them into boxes for my next visit. I can never quite be sure of a client's enthusiasm a week later, because sometimes they only go along with me to be friendly. But the arrangement sticks. Next week I collect my clients in the car and we load it with five boxes of clothing. The three of us beam with pride in the neighbourhood centre as we hand the clothes to Nancy. We stay for a chat and a coffee. Nancy says she is glad to see my clients again. She talks about her work and ambitions for the neighbourhood centre. She says that she would love to attract many more locals in, but is still wondering how it could be done. She is thinking of offering regular meals.

My client's partner says that he is a chef and was in charge of a restaurant long ago. He would love to help with the meals. His wife is enthusiastic and would also love to get involved with the project. We have a lovely chat, and my clients get a sense that this community worker sees them as co-workers. Two days later I get a call from my client to tell me that she approached a lady on the street who appeared to be wandering aimlessly. The lady told my client that she was indeed just wandering around, as her husband had died six months ago. She felt very lost. With pride my client tells me that she has invited this lady to the neighbourhood centre when she and her partner do the cooking.

Reflecting on this process, I realise that I had tried to help my clients connect on the basis of friendliness, doing things together, enjoying activities, having satisfying interaction with the support worker there. None of this had really fired them up. But once they thought they could be of signifi-cance to someone else, the sparks began to fly. It came together for me like the pieces of a jigsaw. This couple, who had led successful professional lives until a few years previously, she as a business manager, he as a restaurateur, had lost not just everything they owned, materially and financially, but also their pride. Now that they had crossed a line and become people in need, the dependence was the very thing they could not escape. They refused to be admitted to psychiatric hospitals, where they were mainly perceived as alcoholics. When they ended up in A&E at general hospitals, there too they were seen as problem cases who had got themselves into the mess they were in. They were told, literally, that their misuse of alcohol was a waste of time and resources that would be better spent on people with genuine problems, such as injury or assault. They were not regarded as victims in need of help, as other people are, but alcoholics who were responsible, or rather to blame, for the problems they faced. They felt stigmatised as psychiatric patients, and as addicts on top of that. Along with shame for the position they were in, they were made to feel guilty.

What they appeared to long for, above all else, was a restoration of hon-our. To be seen and accepted as people who could contribute to society in a meaningful way. The truly special thing is that they rediscovered this in some ways through a sense of pride in what they had been: the woman donated the branded clothes she had worn as a business manager, the man rediscovered his professional identity as a chef, through his ability to cook for others who were having difficulties. They were spurred to action by giv-ing help, instead of receiving it. They regained a sense of pride because we treated them as people, and, because, in the second phase of the process, they had become meaningful again to others. They were able to reclaim a place in society, far away from the exclusion and dependence.

> They showed up at the second-hand clothes fair a couple of times after that, and it was a pleasure to see them, among the other ven-dors, happy in the knowledge that they had the best stall.
>
> In later meetings we talked regularly about their menu for the neighbourhood centre. Thoughts of others and thoughts of being meaningful to others had shattered the mirror in which they saw themselves as losers, and it helped them get along with each other better.
>
> Circumstances conspired to bring me back to the ward, so I couldn't be there for the rest of the story. But they did invite me to an evening meal. It was a case manager's farewell, at which I was the guest and they were the host and hostess.

Quartermaking is about rediscovering connections with organisations, pref-erably outside the mental healthcare setting. The process is different, I have found, for every person or organisation the quartermaker contacts. These clients taught me that notions of connection through friendliness and doing things together do not always work. The driver behind my clients' search for connection was the opportunity to do something for someone else. There is nothing odd about that. We all want to be meaningful to others, don't we?

3.2 Recovery Defined

NURSE: How are you?
CLIENT: I'd rather you didn't ask.
NURSE: Why not?
CLIENT: Because it gives me the feeling you think of me as someone with a problem

When visiting different places in different hospitals on the FACT Team, I notice quite a difference in how people with mental ill health are viewed. The traditional diagnostic view often comes with a superior attitude on the part of the healthcare professional. They see themselves as in charge of the inpatients, and they often seem to forget how their own professional-inpatient relationship colours their observations. I once heard a psychiatrist, for example, argue for a longer stay on a locked ward. She had concluded, on the basis of what she described as a 'hypernormal façade concealing a vast emptiness', that a patient was suffering from 'dementia'. I could tell that her observations were off the mark when her subject, a person I was coaching, let it be known that she stayed as strong as she could in this psychiatrist's presence, and showed no emotion, in case the psychiatrist mistook her anger, at having to stay on the locked ward, as a protest against her authority. She was afraid that revealing her emotions would only lengthen the stay. The vast emptiness that the psychiatrist had observed was merely a reaction to her own authoritarian manner with the patient. Once my client was off the locked ward she returned to the happy, friendly woman she had always been. The test for dementia was never carried out, as it had been unnecessary.

Relations between staff members are of the utmost importance in determining how staff handle or ought to handle patients. In vertically aligned teams these relations are extremely hierarchical. Everything is decided by one person at the top, who need not seek the others' advice. This is often the psychiatrist. The rest of the team just implement the decisions. Patients are usually at the very bottom of these hierarchies and have little or no input. Horizontally aligned teams (Dierinck, 2022), on the other hand, rely on all kinds of consultation and input, a method that gives patients a say or some control over the treatment they receive.

To my mind, community-based care is essentially a change in mental healthcare, and, above all, a change in the relationship between the healthcare professional and patient. The classic relationship is that of the expert care provider versus the sick person who needs the care provider if s/he is to recover her/his health. In community-based care, this relationship is abandoned and the inequality is removed. It is about establishing a person-to-person relationship.

There are many definitions of recovery. Wilma Boevink describes it as (free translation) 'building a meaningful life with or without psychiatric issues' (Boevink et al., 2009, pp. 42–54).

The definition used by the HEE (Herstel, Empowerment en Ervarings-deskundigheid team [Recovery, Empowerment and Expertise team) is: (free translation): Recovery is not the same as cure, but means learning to see where your own vulnerabilities and talents lie and using them take control of your life again (Trimbos.nl).

We are all searching for meaning in our lives. For people with mental ill health this may be a difficult task. A healthcare professional who recognises the importance of recovery will concentrate on the client's search for meaning. As a healthcare professional, then, you are a fellow citizen who can be present, above all, throughout another person's search for meaning.

Machteld Huber offers a new definition of health. The WHO definition of health (1948), as 'general well-being': 'Health is a state of complete physical, mental and social well-being and not merely the absence of disease or infirmity', no longer holds. Major changes, such as longer life expectancies and more chronic diseases, have rendered almost everyone sick under the old definition, meaning that everyone would have to be seen as in a continual state of treatment. Hence Huber's new definition: 'the ability to adapt and to self-manage, in the face of social, physical and emotional challenges' (Huber, 2014).

This concept emphasises the potential to be or stay healthy, even in the face of disease. Of equal importance are personal growth and development and the achievement of personal life goals.

Huber divides the new definition of health into six dimensions: bodily functions, mental functions and perception, spiritual/existential dimension, quality of life, social and sociality participation, daily functioning (Huber et al., 2016). The emphasis is on resilience and self-management.

The old definition contributes heavily to the medicalisation of society, in that many are considered sick for much of their lives. It is also said to place people in an almost constant treatment mode, with a view to finding a cure (Huber et al., 2016). This very phenomenon still exists in psychiatry (Delespaul, 2013). https://doi.org/10.26481/spe.20130411pd.

When the nurse asks the client how he is, and he responds by complaining about the question, he is expressing his dislike of the relationship implied. Alfred, who spent a good ten years in the institution, had been transferred to our ward and now lives independently with the nurse's help. He wants his non-reciprocal relationship with the healthcare professional to end. The nurse asked the question as she would a friend, but the client, still touchy about the ten-year relationship, would rather steer clear of questions that bring it to mind. It will probably take some time for him to appreciate the innocence of the question. The nurse merely used it to start a conversion, as you do when you talk about the weather. The nurse, who actually understands and respects the novelty of the client's situation, makes a mental note not to ask again. In this sense, this man's recovery is also a recovery from his long-term, dependent relationship as an inpatient.

The words 'health', 'cure' and 'treatment' seem to go together. 'Cure' and 'treatment' refer to doctor and patient, but, more particularly, the doctor-patient relationship. The doctor is attributed expertise, the knowledge with which to cure the patient. In this sense, the patient relies on the doctor's knowledge to take him/her forwards and undergoes treatment (Delespaul, 2013). The relationship is based on inequality and dependence. The new definition tells us that health is also about meaningfulness, and that this is something that comes from within. It is not imposed from outside, but something that drives him/her, that makes him/her look forward. It is about self-management. Taking the reins yourself. There will always be situations in which the doctor is the expert who advises treatment to obtain a cure, but, in other circumstances, when cure is not the aim, the new definition causes a shift in the relationship between healthcare professional and patient. When working on patient health, healthcare professionals must ensure that those in need of help are able to self-manage wherever possible. Essentially, then, healthcare is about empowering the client, about being mindful of his/her vulnerability and about safeguarding his/her independence. The new definition of health moves away from the unequal relationship so typical of medicine, towards one in which, above all else, the healthcare professional is of real service.

The professional's attitude is based on the practice of presence. It is about the human dimension, about being there and paying attention (rather than speed and economies of scale), about deep-rooted connection, harmony and a real-life focus (rather than bureaucratic logic), about an attitude of care in the full sense of the words (rather than professionalism), about calm and trust (rather than rapid, results-based interventions), about being an accountable and approachable helper, and about having a belief in the weakest people. When practising the presence approach a worker stays with a person, even if there is no remedy to hand or all remedies have been exhausted. (free translation) 'It is not so much about scoring and problem-solving as searching together for a satisfactory relationship to life – whether that life succeeds, runs aground or comes to an end'. (...) 'The practise of presence (...): it is particularly well suited to people who are difficult to reach (care avoiders, intervention care)' (Baart and Carbo, 2013, pp. 12–13).

Supreme professionalism and humanitarian care go hand in hand. The healthcare professional makes him/herself available as a human being, in a way that allows the client to reveal his/her vulnerability but opens the door to empowerment. Most important of all, the practice of presence must involve a concept of care that allows for vulnerability of the carer, a concept that could easily be discarded in a world where power and authority are key. It always rests on the relationship between the healthcare professional and the person with mental ill health. It is about connecting, attempting to understand something particular, attempting to rediscover what is important and meaningful, and it is often done through exploration, by travelling the road together, precisely because the person with mental ill health is often unable to identify it alone. This way of doing things calls for a type of being there.

Peer supporters are often the best at being there. When connecting through their life stories or personal experiences they can show that they too have encountered what the patient is describing (Campos et al., 2014, 41(2), pp. 49–55). Presence also implies empathy and insight into the suffering of others, through an examination of this suffering and its causes and effects in relationship terms. In the first place, you listen to the client's explanation of how s/he is affected by her/his relationships. You also consider how these problems might affect her/his relationships when s/he is psychotic, for example. When having severe hallucinations a person often seems to fall apart. The primary and most common effect is that, through the nightmare s/he is experiencing, s/he loses all contact with others and ends up in social isolation. The most important thing of all is to restore contact with at least one person, the therapist who wants to be present. The therapist attempts to build a relationship of trust, based on a loving and caring attitude, and, in the second phase, to restore contact between the patient and her/his friends and relatives. In these talks, we absolutely do not go looking to apportion blame for things that have gone wrong, as it were. We try to bring people back together. These two elements: trusting contact between the client and the healthcare professional, and trust between the client and her/his friends and relatives are the foundations for the rest of the work. This is possible only by maintaining presence. Psychiatrists such as Daniel B. Fisher, Peter Breggin and Loren R. Mosher (Mosher et al., 2004) believe that people with severe symptoms of psychosis are capable of recovery, even without medicine. If a healthcare professional is of the opinion that a client should take medication, a refusal cannot be a reason to exclude treatment. Contact can actually bring about a situation in which medication is accepted.

Trying things out with the client, doing things together, creates a tight bond. If things go wrong, you can always grieve or feel sad together. I have experienced this very intensely on several occasions. When a healthcare professional and client can share their sadness about something that hasn't worked out, a stay on a locked ward can be avoided. The bond between healthcare professional and patient makes it possible to overcome crises without force or pressure. 'Bearing it together' alleviates the sadness, which would only escalate to the point of crisis if borne in solitude.

Heather Plett talks about 'to hold space for someone'.

> It means that we are willing to walk alongside another person in whatever journey they're on without judging them, making them feel inadequate, trying to fix them, or trying to impact the outcome. When we hold space for other people, we open our hearts, offer unconditional support, and let go of judgement and control.
>
> Healthcare professionals themselves need the presence of others to enable them to continue working: Sometimes we find ourselves holding space for people while they hold space for others. (...) It's virtually impossible to be a strong space holder unless we have others who will **hold space** for us. Even the strongest leaders, coaches, nurses, etc., need to know that there are some people with whom they can be vulnerable and weak without fear of being judged.
>
> (http://heatherplett.com/2015/03/hold-space/)

Being there and using the relationship as a remedy is certainly a feature of Open Dialogue (ed. Putman and Martindale, 2021).

The most important element in this approach is that of connecting, especially with people who are in deep crisis or psychosis. People lose contact with each other and suffer as a result of this loss. Open Dialogue is about establishing contact without force or pressure. It is not so much a therapy as an attitude that produces an effect. An attitude, as a preliminary to therapy.

3.3 Citizenship and Reciprocity as a Part of Recovery

The wish to live a meaningful life, as expressed by people with mental ill health, has a lot to do with citizenship. Like everyone else, people who have spent a long time in in-patient care long for better social relations and social integration. The idea of citizenship usually rests on some form of reciprocity, and citizenship is thought to occur automatically when people come into contact (ed. Marita Törrönen et al., 2019). You go to work, you get paid. In other words, you do something for someone else, or in the general interests of society, and you receive something in return. You give your neighbour a hand when he moves, later he does something for you. You go shopping for the elderly lady next door and she repays you with a gift. Volunteers get work satisfaction when someone thanks them for their efforts. People take care of each other, and this creates connections.

For some people, however, it does not come automatically. Unable to reciprocate, many are in danger of falling behind. They are seen as scroungers, people on benefits who profit from the goodwill of others and never give anything back. Reciprocity doesn't come easy and so they drop out as citizens too: (free translation) 'If care in the community is be taken seriously, we need to question the citizenship model, as this model gives only those that resemble the standard person the chance to exercise their rights as a citizen to the full' (Kal, 2001, p. 154).

In *Frontiers of Justice* (2007), Martha Nussbaum talks about a citizenship that has no room for people with physical and mental disorders and disabilities. She argues for a different citizenship and suggests a 'capability approach', which rests on a set of social rights, essential to a dignified life. These rights have much in common with human rights. Nussbaum would like to see people belong, even if the system of mutual benefit does not accommodate them and they are in danger of falling behind. Nussbaum is credited with presenting the citizenship model in a way that sets it apart from the idea of normality, which sees reciprocity as an essential, automatic human interaction. Indeed, in Nussbaum we see the spirit that also resides in recovery: it is both craftsmanship and a social movement designed to emancipate and improve the client's lot (Dröes en Van Weeghel, 1994). Contact with peers is an extremely important aspect of this.

Although many people with mental health issues find it difficult to build reciprocal relationships, they often have a strong desire to do so. This is also the case for psychiatric inpatients. If, as a healthcare professional, you are genuinely there for people, they will want to do something in return. But many training courses advise against reciprocal arrangements and may even signal them as an obstacle to a treatment's success, through 'countertransference' (De Witte en Van Dartel, 2019). Healthcare professionals in psychiatric institutions often decline reciprocity. The citizenship model is forced to give ground to the medical model, which is based on distance and inequality. I think that many of us have been trained not to accept gifts from psychiatric patients. For, if we did, it is thought that the patients would be in a position to take advantage. But, given the importance of reciprocity, the acceptance of a gift is merely one way to restore the balance.

3.4 Psychiatry and Social Perspective

In *History of Madness* (2009) Michel Foucault gives us the date of 1657. This year, as he sees it, marks the beginning of the Great Confinement. It is when the *Hôpital Général* in Paris was built. The hospital was founded to deal with the problem of social misfits. Now beggars, vagabonds, criminals and alcoholics could be confined, along with the insane. With this began the reign of reason over irrationality, over chaos. Confinement went hand in hand with a condemnation of laziness, idleness. Madness was deprived of its liberty and constrained. The great confinement largely took place in the second half of the nineteenth century. The strange thing is that psychiatry traces its scientific origin to 'moral treatment', yet there is nothing scientific about this. Foucault says that psychiatric knowledge rested not so much on the moral discourse of the time but on the disciplinary measures available.

> What we call psychiatric practice is a certain moral tactic contemporaneous with the late eighteenth century, which is preserved in the rituals of life in asylums, covered over by the myths of positivism.
>
> (Foucault, 2009, p. 630)

At the time when psychiatry stakes its claim as a science it also happens to be a social and political phenomenon with no apparent regard for the exclusion and isolation of the lunatic. One of the exceptions here is John Conolly, a English contemporary of Pinel's, who complains of exclusion in as early as 1830: 'Once confined, the very confinement is admitted as the strongest of all proofs that a man must be mad (...)' (Conolly, 1830, p. 4).

> shocked and affrighted, he may relapse into his madness and be lost. Or, if his mind has recovered more power, he may understand that he is surrounded by mad people – the raving, the abandoned, the miserable; that his friends have given him up; that he is written in the list of men degraded from the possession of reason, and that he may continue to be confined forever (...) the chances against his perfect restoration are fearful.
>
> (Conolly, 1830, p. 19)

A long stay in a psychiatric institution has a negative effect on a person's self-worth, as a result of the exclusion. Without appropriate help and the intercession of healthcare professionals this becomes a vicious circle, and it is still not easily broken.

Franco Basaglia (1924–1980), whom many associate with the antipsychiatry movement, drew on Conolly to highlight psychiatry's spurious claims to science and its sociopolitical aspect. Basaglia and his allies saw Conolly as a front-runner in the development of the therapeutic community, as set up by Maxwell Jones:

> The classic therapeutic community, set up after 1949 by Maxwell Jones, is based on some key elements: freedom of expression, the destruction of authoritarian relationships, an understanding of the real world, permissiveness, democratization – these are all crucial aspects of the unmasking of asylum structures, which are founded on authoritarian structures, violence, the objectization of the ill patient, the absence of communication.
>
> (Foot, 2015, pp. 108–109)

Ultimately, Basaglia criticised the development of the therapeutic community itself, along with the institutional psychotherapy that grew in France. Yes, it was a process of democratisation from within psychiatry, but they felt that it had not gone quite far enough. While institutional psychotherapy frames the problem in similar terms – inequality of staff/patient relations in a hierarchical structure, insufficient input, greater tolerance, greater fellowship – and emphasises the social fabric... it still places the organisation's needs over those of the resident. Foudraine, in the Netherlands, took a similar view. If a ward was thrown into chaos, for example, they would begin by restoring the peace, not by acting in the residents' interests. The priority, in the end, was always the organisation's ability to function effectively, because without the organisation the patients could not be treated. In the case of environment therapy, patients were eventually treated in a way that kept them living in the organisation (Foot, 2015, p. 318). But if their aim was to stay in the organisation they would not develop fully. Basaglia failed to see the wholesomeness of creating an artificial environment in the institution, outside the community:

> the dangers of escaping into a kind of existential consciousness which would lead to a new objectification. There is an illusion here that you can somehow 'leave the game', and attempt to create a non-organized organisation which is outside of the world of 'power' and its institutions.
>
> (Foot, 2015, p. 120)

They argued that 'there is no such thing as 'outside the system'' (Ibid., p. 121) 'they' refers to Basaglia's supporters.

In the end, Basaglia would advocate the abolition of the psychiatric institution. A statement by a psychiatric reformer in Perugia (Italy) actually seems to refer to what we now call quartermaking:

> At the end of the 1960s the ideology of the good hospital came to an end. A new era opened up – that of the "good territory" (Ibid., p. 246)

"Good territory" could be taken to mean 'welcoming places' in the community.

I see Basaglia as one of the greats of the initiators of the consumer/survivor movement (Oaks, 2006).

His democratic psychiatry sought to reform psychiatry, but, in his fight against exclusion, he himself went much further by placing a question mark over psychiatry altogether; the psychiatric institution is actually a means by which exclusion can be achieved. The movement is also dubious about psychiatry as a science. By aligning itself with the positive sciences, psychiatry felt no obligation to examine its social and societal context: a cover for the need to isolate the psychiatric patient on the basis of words like 'normal' and 'abnormal', 'sick' and 'healthy'.

Basaglia did not go as far as some anti-psychiatrists in ignoring mental health problems and glorifying or romanticising them. This romantic image of 'the good sick person' as opposed to 'the bad society' (environment, provision of care, medical mindset, family, etc.) failed in his eyes to acknowledge the suffering of the person and produced an oversimplified contrast between good and evil. In their romanticisation of psychosis, for example, some psychiatrists went as far as to take hallucinogens to achieve this blessed state and undertake a journey of purification. It did not do them any good. (free translation) 'Anti-psychiatry's reliance on unsupportable claims became ever clearer in the Seventies, even to Laing himself. The "trip" to the depths of madness was good to do. The journey back, to the reborn self, turned out to be much harder' (Hovius, 2013, p. 229).

Basaglia worked in a psychiatric hospital and rejected the 'anti-psychiatry' label. But he can certainly be seen as an anti-psychiatrist if we accept the following definition of the anti-psychiatry movement: (free translation) 'In essence antipsychiatry arises from the meaning in which psychiatry itself is considered part of the problem' (Double, 2002, p. 235).

In describing Basaglia's work John Foot uses the term 'critical or radical psychiatry' (Foot, 2015, p. 44).

If Basaglia was already arranging patient and staff meetings in the institution, as prescribed by institutional psychotherapy, they were not based on workshops or what these workshops should entail, but on the difference between professional and patient roles, and on patient exclusion. In other words, his analysis always covered a person's social and societal position as a patient and the sociopolitical aspect of psychiatry.

When it came to community-based care, Basaglia was also highly alert to evolving power relations between staff and patients. There was always the risk that the unequal patient-professional relationship would persist through the deinstitutionalisation process, and that, systemically, nothing would change. Control mechanisms would develop in new ways in community-based care, requiring people with mental ill health to continue to adapt to society's standards and values. Even in the case of community-based mental healthcare, people with mental ill health would remain shackled.

We see similar concerns in Doortje Kal's work on quartermaking (Kal, 2001). As she sees it, people with mental ill health should not have to integrate by adapting to society, but society should respect diversity and, when needed, adapt to the person with mental ill health.

With every step to a so-called greater humanitarianism, Basaglia remains alert to the systemic aspect of the staff-patient relationship. Psychiatrists and other healthcare professionals view their ability to question their attitude towards people with mental ill health as vastly more important than the 'greater humanitarianism' expressed in 'liberation from chains' and 'breaking free of the institution'. This is because the 'humanitarian' aspect of this apparently growing liberation may actually camouflage the absence of any criticism over the relationship between the psychiatrist and the person with psychiatric issues. Basaglia and his team also understood the paternal dimension that would persist in their work if they practised in the same way outside the institution (Foot, 2015, p. 120).

When psychiatry posits that a subject can be observed scientifically, it does not account for the place in which the observation takes place, i.e. the institution; nor does it account for the institution's effect on the subject under observation. For that reason, its observations frequently confirm initial suspicions: that the best place for the patient is the institution. Whereas, in fact, all that the subject is doing is resisting exclusion, in an attempt to regain control. If the cognitive sciences do not see themselves in a political and social context, they risk being used to exclude or justify the exclusion of the mentally ill. Whereas religion sought to control people through a moral definition of good and evil, the cognitive sciences seek control by defining normality and abnormality.

In psychiatry, people have begun to believe that we must try new ways but that force and pressure will stay necessary (Detombe, 2022). A very pessimistic view. This is precisely why it is important to show that things can be done differently, provided we have the courage to try and are willing to turn existing systems on their heads or, if needs be, replace them. This is what Basaglia demonstrated in Italy.

3.5 The Patient Perspective

Having considered the great confinement, 'moral treatment', the medical model and the therapeutic community, it is time to turn our attention to the patient perspective. This, as shown earlier in this chapter, is all about meaningfulness and the degree of control a person has over their life. When a person is admitted, the main thing is to try to understand how they feel about the admission and how they view their situation. We should also listen to the dreams they once had, as well as their dreams for the future. Have those dreams changed between admissions? How is the change understood? It is important for the professional and the patient, together, to embark on a journey and fulfil at least some of these dreams. Healthcare professionals need to join patients in their search to rediscover their past, present and individuality.

It is important to stop thinking in terms of the resource, and to start thinking in terms of the resource user, be it the patient or the client.

We should look at the side effects of medication (weight gain, reduced activity, etc.) the dynamics of an admission and its accompanying side effects, such as isolation from family and friends, loss of control, etc. We often note that long-stay patients have lost the sense of a future outside the institution, and this is usually down to a loss of hope.

As a healthcare professional at work in an organisation, I assume that you can always develop this patient perspective from within the organisation. But peaceful coexistence will always take precedence over the interests of the individual.

If we consider the ward rules from the patient perspective, for example, we see that they are not always about recovery, but a necessary part of regulating life on the ward, primarily with a view to safety and reducing risks. The rules required by the organisation are not automatically important to the individual.

This applies to my ward, as it does in all organisations. We understand that an inpatient should be allowed to drink alcohol, but that alcohol would be a temptation for a fellow patient who is trying to abstain. In that case, not drinking is a label of respect for others who have problems with alcohol. Aggression on the ward is another issue that affects the safety of others. It disrupts communal life. Only in an emergency will we discharge a person prematurely, if the violations make living with others impossible or certain organisational aspects have genuinely become unworkable. In the case of a discharge, we are still concerned with the individual in line with the 'continuity of care' principle. We look for other ways to accommodate her/him, and s/he may be monitored as an outpatient, either at the organisation or by people from the organisation.

Wandering the corridors aimlessly. Popping into the nurses' station. Quick bike rides between the hospital and the corner shop. Smoking a cigarette at the entrance. Sitting alone among the empty seats in the common room, zapping the TV channels. A closed door, concealing a meeting of healthcare professionals. Telephones ringing. Staff dashing off to deal with an incident on another ward. All part and parcel of life in a psychiatric hospital. With regularity, I hear visitors to psychiatric hospitals describe this as bleak and depressing.

As a healthcare professional you can choose to roam the corridors or sit in the common room, as the patients do, which makes you seem very approachable, but only briefly... because the approachability you create by sitting there locates you in ward time. Discussions on the ward are often brief, because other people wander in and out, talking. The conversation you were originally having with the person sitting there tends to evaporate when others join in. Interference can cloud any real meeting of the minds.

But getting around the ward in this way can be just the right thing to improve the lives of the patients as a whole. Eating at the same table is very important too. This type of presence, sitting around in the common room, may be very necessary, especially if tensions are running high on the ward. It may even be necessary if there is a threat of violence, to allow you to step in quickly and prevent tensions from escalating. Time spent assuring a peaceful environment is essential organisation time.

When patients are difficult to converse with, just sitting around in the common room can be a good way to develop contact. A brief and casual conversation creates a little trust. A momentary encounter in the corridor brings people closer. A good way to get yourself noticed is to invite the patient in.

Your colleagues are on the ward, and you see them at briefings, transfers, team meetings, intervision sessions and work meetings. They even hold you back at times. Just being a member of staff keeps you busy. Often, you have the feeling that everything is coming at you, and not that you are making headway. You are inundated with conversations, it seems, and they too are constantly interrupted by everyone else who wants to talk to you. My colleagues and I are like the pivotal point of the ward, around which the others revolve. A symbolic hub, the nurses' station, marks the difference between 'us' and 'them'. It marks the boundary.

Working on a ward as I do, I know that a ward can restrict a recovery-based approach. I know that a psychiatric ward has a dynamic that you, the healthcare professional and the team, must resist if you aim to relate to a patient properly. The dynamic exists even when the team has the very best intentions and makes every conceivable effort to be there for its patients. To begin with, you need to be aware of this dynamic, to know that it also affects you, not because you are wrong about people, but precisely because you work on a ward. As healthcare professionals, we are often busy with all kinds of things, but our fatigue at the end of the day is not really an indicator of the work we put into our patients; because a lot of our time goes into the organisation. It is important to maintain a counter dynamic, focused on greater control for the patient and more room and space outside the institution. The dynamics of the institution can make you put your own organisation ahead of patient time. Team meetings, briefings, work meetings, intervision sessions, colleague support... all of which take up organisation time, which you hope is to the benefit of the patients now. But you cannot be entirely certain. Patients frequently complain that staff are too busy attending meetings. I cannot say they are wrong.

It is important to arrange your time so that the majority is spent in patient time. This means setting time aside to talk to patients individually, and regularly. In the patient's home, I am the visitor and automatically in his/her time. At home, s/he takes centre stage. S/he is the one in control. In my three years on the FACT Team, on home visits, I have experienced how different this is to the work I was accustomed to on the ward. When visiting a home I am someone else's guest. The knock at the door is not for me, but the person I have come to visit. I have brief encounters with other visitors who are not there for me, but for the same reason as me. Home visits involve my being increasingly in my clients' lives, and additional encounters with important people in each client's world are often major elements of my work. When I see people in their homes I often sense a certain loneliness, but an ordinary kind of personal loneliness, not the loneliness marked by a stay in an institution or community, where everyone experiences the same solitude whether they know each other or not. The dynamic of the institution seems to inhabit the walls, the windows, the furniture. No matter how colourful they may be, they seem only to suggest a sad fate when the people staying there are in for a long time.

> (free translation) The patient is living in asylum time, isolated, and the family has already spent years living without him or her. But they do think about their son or daughter constantly. We, the care providers, have our time with our colleagues. These are three different, entirely separate times. Each makes their own way through this time, and their own way through life. In rehabilitation psychiatry, the art is to dedicate yourself to establishing a little synchronicity between the three parties, not just theoretically but very specifically by thinking that a boy has a mother who is thinking about him, and that a care provider could give her a call now and then, even when things are going well. As a care provider you can adjust your own time, through all the stress and notes and reorganisations, to how the patient and his family live their time. Even if time is short through a shortage of staff, this synchronisation of the times is vital, because it is precisely that which gives someone a sense that life is changing again.
>
> (Petry, 2011, p. 61)

Healthcare professionals spend much of their time applying ward rules, which are vital to the quality of ward life, but ward time and patient time are different things.

> Alphons doesn't wash up. For a while now he has been irritating fellow patients and staff. The weekly washing-up rota agreed by the patients doesn't seem to work. The kitchen is in a disorganised state. It comes up repeatedly in staff briefings, and we keep hearing of people's dissatisfaction with it. Some staff even sigh at the mention of his name. Soon, he will get the blame for every mess in the kitchen. People are beginning to react to him, and the situation is getting edgy.
>   He does his own cooking. It's a beautiful thing to behold. He creates a speciality dish and takes pride in it. He gives his assigned nurse a taste, and she savours the moment with him. Little things like this create a bond with him. He is pleased with his culinary skills, glad his assigned nurse appreciates them. Yet, for the sake

of organisation, because he won't wash up, it looks like being over-shadowed. In the briefings and team meeting his assigned nurse speaks about the importance of the cooking. She won't go along with the idea of banning him from the kitchen because he leaves it in a mess. She understands the washing up issue, the irritation of staff and patients, and she raises the matter with him. He says he has taken it on board, and retires to his room after cooking... without washing up. His assigned nurse has every faith that he will do as asked. She speaks to her colleagues about the arrangement she has made with him. Her colleagues agree to ask the patients for patience if they complain about the mess, and, above all, not to clean it up. And so the kitchen stays in a mess. The assigned nurse passes the message to the new shift, the night staff. And, in the morning, after yet another shift has ignored the mess, and his fellow patients have again shown restraint, he cleans the kitchen. Colleagues and fellow patients are pleasantly surprised. The assigned nurse has pushed organisation time aside to allow for the individual time of a patient who likes to cook. It took some doing. She made certain her colleagues got the picture, and they in turn took the trouble to explain it to complaining patients and win them over. It took time and effort to safeguard this individual time. Room for individual time comes at a heavy cost to organisational time, but is worth the effort. He cooks and enjoys it. It raises his self esteem. One way to prioritise the organisation would have been to ban cooking after a certain time. A rule of that type would have ensured a smooth-running organisation and a tidy kitchen. It would have been a decision in the interests of the group, the organisation, and not the individual. In the long term, however, the assigned nurse's actions showed fellow patients that, given time, he would actually tidy the kitchen. So he was back in their good books.

We need to be aware that a ward is run in organisation time, not individual time. To make room for individual time you push organisation time aside, and it takes a lot of work: making individual arrangements, conveying them to incoming colleagues on the next shift, convincing them to stick with these arrangements and interact with other patients on this basis. Hardly the path of least resistance. Grouping people by their progress through a course of treatment can sometimes lead to strange organisational leaps. Additional groups, with wonderful-sounding names, are sometimes created to spare an organisation's blushes after failure. An 'observation group', in which nothing actually happens, is a handy way to paper over the cracks. In the really quite hopeful book, *Depressief. Goede zorg voor kwetsbare mensen* (2014), Hans Meganck writes of his admission to a psychiatric hospital. He spends two weeks in group 0, an observation group, where nothing is done with him. It turns out that there was no room in the therapy group, and the observation group was set up while he waited for a place. He gets nothing from this and feels that nobody is concerned with him. Patients have high expectations, and rightly so, when they admit themselves to a psychiatric hospital. It is not something you take lightly. If most of the time is spent waiting, for organisational reasons, you feel not just disappointed, but cheated. In *Psychotic mum: An inside story* (2019) Brenda Froyen describes her expectation that her issues will be addressed at the point of involuntary admission. She expects the healthcare professionals to be there for her, especially when she is restrained. It does not happen. She feels left to her fate. We might suppose that an organisation does a truly great job if its healthcare professionals are given every opportunity and incentive to be there for a patient outside the organisation's time. It may sound strange, but a patient's individual time, the time that truly aids her/his progress, has to be almost wrestled from organisation time, the time that yields nothing for her/him. From this perspective, it is important for an organisation to allow a little slack in its rules and regulations. As a healthcare professional you can be so busy that most of your time is spent on immediate problems. Giving medications, making breakfast, waking patients, ticking boxes, opening and closing room doors for patients, helping to solve minor everyday conflicts, taking people to therapy sessions, getting people to participate in therapies, making observations, attending briefings, team meetings, intervision sessions, work meetings... Your presence is vital when it comes to managing the ward and getting everything to run smoothly. That is just how it is. But you should realise that this is time as experienced by the healthcare professional, not time as experienced by the patient, or the patient's friend or relative. I hear patients say to staff, 'You're here from eight to five. We're here all the time, and that's a whole other experience'. The mere fact of being always there, sometimes day and night, with staff in and out in waves, produces a very different perspective. To create an opening, to synchronise organisation and personal time, you have to be aware of the difference in the first place. Only then can you tackle the difference. Willingness to listen and empathy are key. You step out of your own perception of time, which is bound up with the ward and your organisation, and into the patient's perception of time.

Below therapy programmes there is another layer of time: the anniversary. We are used to celebrating the anniversaries of good things: a year older, a new year beginning, a wedding anniversary. We are less public in our remembrance of the painful events in our lives. There are no printed verses in cards to mark the fifth anniversary of a loved one's passing, yet sympathy is just as important at those times. We like to consider these things on the ward, and when patients first arrive we ask them to tell us the dates of difficult days (the anniversary of a parent's death, the anniversary of a child's death, the birthday of a significant person...), and we ask what to do when those dates come around: start a conversation about a birthday, perhaps, or just give a little more of our time without mentioning it explicitly. The anniversary date and the patient's instructions for the staff are then recorded in the ward's electronic diary, which only the staff can read. All staff check the diary when they start their shift, so the arrangements are always seen on the day. Many patients are reassured to know that we understand the importance of this date. They feel much less alone in their sadness just knowing it. A freeze on patient time often corresponds with a boost in organisation time. Another dynamic on the ward is that staff tend to freeze a patient's time just when things are going well for her/him. When s/he is stable and ready for change s/he is advised against it, encouraged to hold on tight to his hard-won stability. Healthcare professionals are often aware of the risk that change can bring. They may advise a person not to do something to spare them the disappointment of further failure. Does the healthcare professional tend to keep things as they are because s/he is afraid that the work will have been in vain? An overly sensitive care reflex protects the patient from disaster, but protects against change. This can deny someone a part of what defines them as a human being: the longing for change, the longing for renewal...

As human beings we are marked by the passage of time, and the flow of time brings change. It is better, I think, to let people experience loss than freeze time to avoid it. Knowing that you will be there in times of momentous loss is what gives people the courage to live. They know that you cannot always be there for them, and that they will have to manage on their own once they are discharged, once outpatient therapy ends, but that they can also call on you if the going gets hard. The coach is someone who walks alongside you and maintains a presence. He/she is not some pandering, conservative guardian who constantly fends off failure. No one should be protected from misfortune or loss. In this manner, people regain the courage to manage their lives.

The client should always be able to see a healthcare intervention as supportive. S/he should take a healthcare professional's feedback, or criticism, as the basis for consultation. The intervention should allow room for authentic cooperation between patient and healthcare professional.

At talks, people sometimes comment that I only ever mention the success stories. I say that, with my method, success stories are all I know, because I stay present with my clients and their goals, and I am there when things go wrong. There is no such thing as failure if failures are shared. My guaranteed presence is the success. The presence is the success, and as a healthcare professional this is usually in your own hands.

As well as stepping out of organisation time, and into patient and family time, you can allow the client to break into organisation time. You can reduce meetings without clients to a minimum. Clients attend team meetings when it is they who are under discussion. Most are suspicious, the first time around. Until now, they have only been invited when things are going badly. They suspect they are in for a telling-off. But when that turns out not to be the case, and they leave feeling that there is a team behind them, they have a strong sense of support. Clients, even the more introverted ones, have been known to speak up unexpectedly at one of these meetings and to thank everyone for being there. This is always a very special moment for me.

A team meeting involving a patient, colleagues and other significant people, such as family and friends, is time-consuming from an organisational point of view. When it is just you and your colleagues, many more clients can be discussed. The time this saves is often just an illusion. When decisions are needed, team meetings often culminate in a compromise between the various healthcare professionals present. If the client is not there, compromises reached in this way can turn out to be inadequate, because some important client information will have been overlooked. We end up holding the meeting again. A team meeting without a client produces all kinds of hypotheses, which are often swept away when the patient is present. With the client there the quality of the meeting is better, and in the long run it saves on organisation time.

Team meetings involving the client are particularly good when the client gets to pick the team. In that case, the people closest to him/her, who know him/her best, are present. A wonderful coincidence of organisation time and client time. A meeting of this kind makes the client's suffering more expressible, especially for the client. A house of words can be built, which the client is happy to inhabit.

> We have just taken a group photo of the people who were at this exceptional meeting: his team. Claude himself occupies a chair at the front, entirely at ease. At his side, a friend and her husband. They have known him for ten years or more. It is unusual for people to have been around for so long, given that he drifts from one place to another, from street to temporary accommodation, to a bed in a psychiatric hospital. I am seeing them for the first time. On the other side, the peer supporter who works on our team. Lately she has been out with him regularly. He has given her his life story. She has spoken about her own issues. When talking to him there are always silences, which you, the healthcare professional, can best fill with references to what you see and hear around you, or often just a few words about yourself. He always checks back into the conversation, even if just with a smile. He says that he is suffering, but can't say much more about it. He has this one little phrase for the healthcare professionals: 'I'm having a hard time.' But if you insist on knowing what he means by it, the conversation dries up instantly. He wants someone to be there, but without having a real conversation. Lyotard would speak of 'inexpressible suffering' (Held, 2005). I stand behind him in the photograph, alongside a

psychiatrist from a former admission at another psychiatric unit. He was keen to have her at the meeting. She listened to him and got to know him very well. She has arranged the meeting in a room at her hospital. The man who took the photo is a trainee peer supporter. He is on an introductory placement on our ward. He doesn't know Claude, but in response to Claude's story he has spoken about himself and his own experiences at the meeting. Claude feels supported by this man's presence. "The more the merrier", he adds with a laugh. We see the meeting as a party, a gathering of people who are well disposed towards him. He knows that they will not unite to pull the wool over his eyes, or suggest anything he wouldn't want to go along with. This is exactly what he needs. People he can talk to, although he says so little. Even I, the organiser, feel like a visitor on foreign soil, here at his former psychiatrist's hospital. She tells us what Claude was like on his previous stay. She speaks of a person who hears voices, can be psychotic and uses alcohol to self-medicate. He needs to be in a relationship, like everyone else, but often ends up with women who take advantage, and then runs into financial difficulties. His tremendous isolation makes him vulnerable to exploitation by others. The psychiatrist talks about his loneliness, which is often too hard to bear.

Claude nods in response to this account. He tells his former psychiatrist about his present situation, and says that he has stopped using alcohol and that, for his own protection, he is not currently in a relationship. By giving an account of how things used to be the psychiatrist has unwittingly thrown Claude's present efforts into sharper focus. The difficulties he has had and his efforts to deal with them were not addressed on his current admission. He is proud to have changed his approach to life. The psychiatrist nods in admiration. His friend speaks about how she met Claude after being admitted to a psychiatric hospital herself. She says that they always have stayed in touch. She talks about how he used to live. I speak about Claude's current admission, and the efforts he is making. I mention Claude's past and the death of his father, who couldn't handle the divorce. Claude was eleven at the time. His mother was disinterested in him and neglected him badly. He was forced to fend for himself. Claude's woes began with his father's death. It marked the beginning of a kind of odyssey, which has never ended. The peer supporter from our team adds a few details that she has picked up from her conversations with Claude. It seems that we are here at this meeting, in his presence, to write his history. Each of us makes a contribution, and together we construct his story. We create in words, so difficult for Claude to find, a shared and understood picture of the past, present and future. The participants add new layers and Claude is given words that he can use. Not words coloured by diagnoses and symptoms, pinned on from the outside in a way that alienates. The suffering, his suffering, is made expressible. It is made comprehensible in relationship terms, made reworkable from a relationship perspective. His plans for the future are shaped by his past. He speaks of his traumatic childhood and desire to leave Flanders, as it constantly reminds him of those terrible experiences. The psychiatrist touches briefly on another patient, who moved because his old house reminded him of the psychotic episodes he had had there. He asks to be admitted when a new psychotic episode threatens, to that his new home isn't tainted by these psychotic experiences. We are aware of the administrator's grave doubts over Claude's plans and accept her request for home support. For the first time ever, he agrees. His friends talk about his former home. From their descriptions we get our first inkling that his landlord was unreliable. A picture emerges of Claude as an unassertive person, who ends up in highly vulnerable situations. With no tenancy agreement in place the landlord found it easy to throw Claude onto the street. This time the preparations will take longer, but the foundations will be much firmer. By providing support at home we may be able to prevent the restlessness that ultimately goes with the brief spells of home living and soon leads to homelessness. Made-to-measure support. We have taken an important step today. It does him a power of good to have all these sympathetic people gathered around him. After the meeting he and I go for a coffee and have another look at the group photo. We digest it all and recap what everyone said.

Claude is obviously traumatised by his childhood experiences. In the documentary *One More Time with Feeling* (2016) the musician Nick Cave speaks about time and trauma:

> Time is elastic. We can go away from the event (the loss of his son). When we move away we're like on a rubber band, and life can go on and on and on, but eventually it just keeps coming back to that thing. And that's some kind of trauma, I guess.

When people are traumatised, the passage of time appears distorted, or at least they experience it very differently. Life goes on after trauma, and you live on, until the elastic snaps you back to the time of the trauma, and it hits you as hard as it did the first time. Time has become elastic, in other words, and the further passage of time seems like an illusion. As a carer for people who have experienced frequent and severe trauma, it is important to understand, accept and move in synch with this passage of time. Visiting a client's family allows you to see how time is experienced by the other significant people in the patient's life. Organisation time is important, because a ward has to function, but it has little to do with the patient's time or the family's time. In fact, organisation time can get in the way of recovery.

On the ward, Ria seems a little disinterested, even flippant. She is not really talking. She is frequently in conflict with her fellow patients. Nurses are having to spend a lot of their energy intervening in these quarrels. Time and again they are having to judge whether she or the others are responsible. The people around her tend to think she is a stirrer. Patients are brought together to talk the hostilities through. Warnings are even issued to the parties concerned. It gets so bad that her admission is under question. We realise that we are dealing with her in what is basically organisation time.

> When we step into her context and out of the ward context we see what is bothering Ria. She tells me that her son has been homeless for months. He usually stays at the night shelter. From what she is telling me, he sounds worn down and embittered. I say that he might need help, and that I am willing to try. We see a deeply dejected son, resentful that others are doing so well while he has lost everything, self-respect included. This is expressed through anger, shouting, destroying his debit card and talking about suicide, immediately, that very day. Ria cries and says no more. Obviously, she can't deal with this alone.
>
> Finding Ria a home is obviously more than simply a practical task. Everything centres on the relationship between mother, son and daughter-in-law. The son still fixates on his mother for help, and she is an inpatient at our centre. He finds it hard to accept help from anyone else. By viewing Ria's housing issue as a family problem, and finding an authority that will also provide assistance for her son and his girlfriend, we can get to work on Ria's housing issue. We take the matter up with the son's healthcare workers. Ria sees our efforts on her family's behalf as support for her. We are helping her to care for her son. The 'healthcare-Ria-family' triangle is essential in establishing a stability of some sort. Through Ria, we can now take the trust she places in the care provision and transplant it to her son's relations with the other healthcare professionals. The support provided for her son reassures her that she can now give her own life a little more consideration. We see a completely different Ria on the ward. Knowing that we supported her in her maternal role, she is much more earnest in her conversations with the healthcare professionals. There are fewer conflicts on the ward and she is openly appreciative of the assistance she was given to help her son. By assisting a patient's family you can rediscover the desires of the patient, such as solidarity with a close relative, despite what are often major family problems. That desire has

become deeply buried, because every attempt the person has made to care for that family member has been fruitless. Offering help for a family member can allow you to rediscover a client's request for support and work with the client independently of what are often less significant dramas on the ward. Fail to discover the request for support and you can become stuck in organisation time, facing a patient who just seems to be hanging around the ward causing trouble.

By focusing on the mother-son relationship we step into patient time and family time. To the outsider, helping Ria's son may seem like a waste of time. It does take a lot of effort: planning a large meeting of healthcare professionals, encouraging the son's original healthcare professionals to take up his case again, reuniting the family and administrators and ultimately, with patience, resolving sky-rocketing tensions through catharsis at the meeting itself. Besides improving the quality of life for all concerned, it saves organisation time in the long run. In the wake of the big meeting we spend less time dealing with conflicts on the ward. The self-harming of the patient also comes to an end, which means and end to the accident and emergency referrals and the stays on the locked ward.

This may be the ideal juncture, before continuing with the patient's time and the organisation's time, to take a closer look at the importance of cooperating with family.

3.6 Family

By introducing experts by experience in Belgium (Article 107) mental healthcare in general has moved away from a conflict model. The relationship between healthcare professionals and patients was essentially one of conflict (Gids naar een betere geestelijke gezondheidszorg, 2002).

The care providers saw the knowledge they possessed as central to patient care. They saw themselves as having the knowledge and expertise to help the patient. If s/he disagreed, this was often put down to the symptoms of the illness, which came in the form of a diagnosis. Therapies were developed to suit the diagnosis, and the patient was made to have therapy (often group therapy) for the diagnosis he was given (Delespaul, 2013). This attitude was a frequent cause of conflict between patients and healthcare professionals as patients often failed to see the relevance of the therapies they were forced to have.

Alongside a relationship of conflict between the healthcare professional and patient, there was often conflict between the healthcare professionals and the people in the patient's immediate environment. Some in the anti-psychiatry movement identified society as the cause of mental illness, and blamed the immediate environment, the parents, for their children's mental health problems (Laing, 1965). Patients were seen as needing to be protected from a debilitating family climate and a society that was generally hostile towards them. Admission and isolation from others were viewed as an opportunity for respite.

When I started out in the field, towards the end of the 1980s, very little attention was given to family, and, when it was, family was presented in a negative light. Relatives who would ask persistent and specific questions about a sick relative were viewed as troublesome, not as folk who were also trying to figure out what was happening to their loved ones. The inconvenience they caused by pressing healthcare professionals for information was perceived by the very same professionals as an indication of how they treated their mentally ill relative, and this 'troublesome' behaviour was applied wholesale as the reason for all the relative's problems. The harder the family pushed for contact, the more the healthcare professionals stressed the need to separate the patient from them. The carers perceived family members as a hindrance, and a restriction to the patient's development. When a family did not ask many questions, that too was seen as the cause of illness. In the end, every conceivable behaviour was interpreted as toxic. This meant that relatives were denied the right to support, unless they were willing to adjust their behaviour in accordance with the professionals' definition of normal. Here too, the healthcare professional came across as all-knowing, as the person in control.

Healthcare professionals widely believed that patients had to be protected from their toxic families. The aim was to isolate the patient, thereby gaining maximum exposure to the healing power of therapy and contact with healthcare professionals. Patients were also prescribed respite from a society that was too demanding and dangerous for them.

A counter movement came through groups that felt mistreated by healthcare professionals. Patients themselves said that healthcare professionals did not listen, and they asked for their views to be taken into account. In Belgium a survivor organisation, Uilenspiegel (Van de Vloet, 2013–2014, p. 4), was formed in 1997, and this organisation squared up to the healthcare profession. A family organisation, Similes, also emerged, and they carried the fight to healthcare professionals, refusing to accept that the finger should be pointed at them, or that their opinions should be ignored. There was also discord between these patient and family organisations (Similes, 2012, p. 5).

By now the conflict model ought to be behind us. On the whole, community-based care aims to view things in contextual terms and to be inclusive of all parties. The new outlook in mental healthcare should help these groups, modelled originally on unions or interest representatives, to bury the hatchet. In community-based care, there is a will to return the management of treatment and recovery to the patient, and a will to see the patient's family and the broader environment as partners in the care (Gids naar een betere geestelijke gezondheidszorg, 2002).

On the ward, we pay proper attention to long-broken family bonds. We find out how the break occurred, and see if there is anything we can do to fix it. We bear in mind that new developments, through circumstances outside our control, can always bring people closer. We work on the idea of 'momentum', or the idea that some – often coincidental – situations or events can create openings that allow us to set up a contact that we did not previously think possible. It can come too late at times. It is an unfortunate but regular occurrence for family members to tell us, at an inpatient's funeral, of their regret at not having been in touch.

As healthcare professionals, we know that repairs of family bonds often elicit a host of conflicting emotions in the people we support, as well as in other family members. There is always the fear of new disappointments, or that a renewal of contact will lead to nothing. Along with the happiness that contact brings there can be painful talks about why family members have been out of touch for so long. People do not always see past events in the same way. We assume that the benefits of renewing contact most certainly outweigh the often temporary difficulties that can arise in the process, and that the support we offer as healthcare professionals is vital in healing the bonds between family members; a process that often takes time and care. We expect renewed contact to bring a temporary imbalance in the patient's state of mind, and we discuss this with them. We assume that there is great strength in the rediscovery of bonds between people who are hugely significant to each other. All-too-often family members have been put off by a string of hopes and disappointments, which have always ended in despair. In many unsupported situations, where bonds with family members have not been pursued, we arrive too late. Relatives appear to have taken respite by distancing themselves from the patient, although this respite is merely relative. The healthcare professional who attempts to heal a long-broken bond will often need a great deal of time, and will need to know that the person he is supporting can remain stable for long enough to give family members the courage needed to build meaningful and sustainable contact.

In *De zorgval* (Baart and Carbo, 2013, p. 35) the relatives of vulnerable people are described as having a 'secondary vulnerability'. Not originally vulnerable in themselves, they have become so as a result of a relative's vulnerability. Marijke Kars (2012), who authored a study on the parents of children with cancer, postulates that the bond, role and responsibilities of parenthood make parents susceptible to a powerful secondary vulnerability.

It is our task as healthcare professionals to identify and understand this secondary vulnerability, and certainly not to exacerbate it. As the person responsible for a relative with mental ill health, a family member can face choices that increase their secondary vulnerability. These choices only ever result in loss. The healthcare professional can prevent this in some circumstances by taking action or decisions on behalf of the mentally ill relative to relieve the family of the burden.

> (free translation) Good care does not force these vulnerable people to decide the "impossible", but requires care providers to summons the humanity and courage to do the difficult work themselves. True acknowledgement of this secondary vulnerability requires acceptance of the fact that you yourself as a care provider have a job to do, rather than may way for the client's self management.
>
> (Baart and Carbo, 2013, p. 41)

In a talk with a mother and son, the mother says that she had her son involuntarily admitted on a couple of occasions. This was at times when he was so psychotic that he was a danger to himself. Her actions have severely clouded the relations between them. He feels that she doesn't trust or believe him and that she has literally taken away his freedom. The mother tells him how hard it was for her to make those decisions. She was watching her son drift off into a world of psychosis, which, although it brought him happiness, came with very great sadness, and most of all fear. She saw him drift deeper into drugs and felt unable to stand by and watch as he put himself in danger. She had him involuntarily admitted. Now that we and her son are reflecting on that time she says she is glad to hear that the healthcare professionals are prepared to look out for him and to take responsibility if he looks like putting his life in danger. We talk to the son about these dangerous situations. The mother says she wants just one thing, and that is to re-establish the bond with her son. Her secondary vulnerability was due to the power she was forced to exercise over her son at the times when he was in danger. She could either do nothing and lose him altogether, or have him committed and end up clashing with him. I often hear parents speak about the decision they made to authorise an involuntary admission, and about how guilty they felt afterwards for acting against that family member's wishes. Those feelings of guilt were only exacerbated by the force that was used to achieve it.

It is best if healthcare professionals take the responsibility for having a known patient admitted involuntarily, if they and the parents or other parties believe this is vital to the safety of the patient or others around them. For the patient and the family, it is extremely important that a voluntary admission be handled with compassion. Excessive force can be traumatic for either or both.

A mother, whose son was regularly aggressive, told us once that things had gone so badly in previous admissions that the healthcare professionals had called to say they were discharging her son, and that she could come and collect him from the locked ward. This telephone conversation was the only contact the healthcare professionals had had with her. The mother could not imagine having her son living at home. His aggressive behaviour was the very reason for his admission. She felt that the service had let her down, twice. Firstly, by not inviting her sooner after his admission, and secondly by putting her in the situation of having to refuse to allow him back home. It felt like having to throw him out again. Here too, the woman had no options, and by making these demands of her the healthcare professionals had only increased her secondary vulnerability. Allowing her son back home would be a source of horrendous difficulty and aggression and refusing him would sour their relationship even more. In circumstances like these, it is up to the healthcare provider to ensure the continuity of the care. Indeed, the patient is entitled to continuity of care. When the organisation runs into serious difficulties, it is the healthcare professional who should find continued support for the patient elsewhere. In this sense, the healthcare professional is best advised to develop a network of organisations through which continuity of care is guaranteed. Turning to parents and relatives is not an option in these cases. It is also very important to consider an inpatient's children. People in in-patient care find it extremely difficult to fulfil their parental role. We observe many negative emotions: guilt and feelings of powerlessness due to the inability to provide appropriate care for the child. This can agitate a parent and produce challenging behaviour on the ward. I often saw healthcare professionals advising a parent on a ward to distance from the child in an effort to bring the patient a sense of calm. But this distance benefits no one: neither the child, nor the inpatient. It is actually up to the healthcare professional to be more present in the search for connection, to be present at visits and to build a bridge between the parent and the child, in agreement with the child's support workers, if there are any. You give the parent hope that everything will be okay. Understandably, this is a process of trial and error. The only assurance you can give is that you will stay present, as a contact, throughout the difficulties. It doesn't seem like much, but it can mean a lot to the patient. It is the only way to make a true connection and render yourself, as the healthcare professional, surplus to requirements in the end.

> The son of Gilbert is in a foster home. There came a time when he couldn't provide a father's protection. He is grateful for everything the foster family does for his son, but is also worried about losing his paternal role. His son is doing very well in his foster family. The father panics at any sign of his son's growing independence and responds with anger and irritation, which makes his son even less inclined to visit. On the ward the father is disheartened, agitated and irritated. The team feels like it is going around in circles. Tensions in the father-son relationship are seen as an obstacle to the father's development, and the team decides that, to restore calm, father and son should not see each other for some time. He accepts this, and his depression deepens. He stops telling the healthcare

76

professionals about his desire to see his son. He talks about the pointlessness of life. Now the healthcare professionals focus even more intently on the depression, and, thinking that this could be a long admission, they refer him to our ward. At rehab we begin by asking what it is that gives him meaning in life, what it is that he finds important, and he finds the courage to mention his son again. We contact the foster support worker and cancel the previous team's arrangements. We pave the way for a meeting between father and son. We try for a relationship that allows Gilbert to rediscover his paternal role, as he is always keen to know what his son is up to. We advise the father not to shower his son with gifts, as the son could interpret this as trying to make up for shortcomings as a father. It works. By the end of the meeting the son is chatting away about his interests. The two become much closer in this initial meeting. Afterwards, in a one-on-one, the father tells me of his love for his son, and his feelings of guilt. A host of new memories and questions arises after this first meeting in six months with his son, and we talk them through at length. This act of repairing family bonds by drawing on the network (the foster care support worker and foster parents) reboots or alters the dynamics of the psychotherapy.

As a healthcare professional it is important to understand that your role in coaching the client is modest and supportive, but that you can take a unique position by addressing both the mental health issues of the patient and the secondary vulnerability of the family.

It is also quite wonderful as a healthcare professional, to collaborate with a family peer supporter. It is interesting to examine this person's position in the team in the context of connection and collaboration.

Our FACT Team decided that in addition to having a lived experience expert for clients, we would have a peer supporter for families. This is a member of staff like the others, but not a professional. Not identical, but on an equal footing with a healthcare professional. The mere fact that he works alongside the team's professionals is a token of our parting with the conflict model in favour of a cooperation or solidarity model (Hopkins, 2021).

He is a care partner in the sense that a client's family members are care partners. We inform and support family members, and, in some cases, try to establish a new balance between them and the client, without allowing either to take precedence. We think in contextual terms and may even try to alter the context to establish equality between the partners. The family peer supporter rises above his own experience, views it dispassionately through his understanding of other relatives' experiences, and so steps beyond his own most individual, personal experiences. By taking this step the family peer supporter rises above himself as a person and listens to the experiences and stories of other family members. From this perspective, the family peer supporter knows when to listen, when to be present and when to share his own experience with family members.

A family peer supporter has learnt not to compartmentalise, not to view mental health in terms of good and bad.

He has learnt to stop apportioning blame for his own family member's mental ill health. The parents of a child with mental ill health may begin by wondering whose genes or behaviours are behind the mental health issues. The family peer supporter is beyond the issue of blame, beyond the sense of injustice about what happened, and, therefore, beyond any victim mentality. He no longer seeks protection from the pain of his experience by finding someone else to blame.

He has strong defences against anyone who comes across as overly sympathetic about what he 'has been through'. He recognises it as a means by which others take the high ground. He has come to this realisation without resentment or envy.

He is aware of the dynamics of suffering. Partners can grow apart when a relative suffers mental illness. They often process their suffering and secondary vulnerability at different rates, and one may have reached acceptance whereas the other has not. This can create tensions between partners. If they are aware of these dynamics, they have a good chance of bridging the gap and maintaining the connection.

To summarise, the family peer supporter has reached a certain level of acceptance of his own family situation. This is not to say that he has stopped thinking about his family situation, or stopped trying to improve the life of his mentally ill relative. The search for improvement does come as a personal defeat to him if results are not immediately forthcoming. He views the search as a process of personal development.

The family peer supporter stays in regular contact with other family peer supporters and shares experiences with them.

The family peer supporter has a wide range of tasks. He supports family members in their search for relaxation and respite, to help them continue to function in a caring role. He checks with the family to see which activities might bring respite. The family peer supporter may also approach clubs and associations in the quartermaker's role. He helps family members break through the isolation they are experiencing. He looks for places where family members can access self-care and draws on his own network of contacts to do so.

If this is not successful, the family peer supporter can recommend a healthcare professional or help find one for family members.

A family peer supporter empowers the family in their communication with staff on the family member's ward.

A family peer supporter meets the mother of a person with mental ill health who complains that the nurses keep fobbing her off by referring her to the monthly talk with the psychologist. She would like to receive information for the family much more often, possibly through her son's caregiver. The family peer supporter advises this family member to ask the psychologist, at the next monthly meeting, to permit her son's assignment nurse to give information more frequently. Family peer supporters often give families advice on the best way to deal with healthcare professionals. Through experience, theirs and that of other peer supporters, family peer supporters have learned the rules that deliver the best chances of getting what you want from healthcare professionals. In this case the family peer supporter advised the family member to be less emotional when speaking to the carers, because they have a strong tendency to label a relative's emotions negatively as 'the family's excessive concern about the ill relative'. A label which makes them less inclined to take the substance of a family's questions seriously, as they are too preoccupied with what they see as overly powerful emotions. And so in this service healthcare professionals tend to fob family members off, rather than deal with their questions. A family peer supporter will also continue to give the family members a positive view of the future. Hope is vital for family members too.

A family peer supporter helps to explain the healthcare professionals' jargon.

But family peer supporters often also signal systematic problems, such as a lack of continuity in the transition from child psychiatry to adult psychiatry.

Family peer supporters may also signal problems to the healthcare professionals and colleagues on their team. They can use information gained from the family to turn attention to the gravity of a mentally ill person's situation, to enable these colleagues to begin working with the client sooner and more intensively. This allows them to bridge the gap between the family and the client's support workers.

The greater the secondary vulnerability of the family members the more important it is for a family peer supporter to attend. There is no one better placed to draw the family's attention to the significance of secondary vulnerability. He can also warn the healthcare professional against a potential increase in secondary vulnerability.

Of interest, there are concerns over the degree to which family peer supporters may seek professional training to gain recognition for what they do. In my experience, not many professionals are not entirely open to the idea of collaborating with family peer supporters (or peer supporters in general). This disdain can give family peer supporters a tendency to prove themselves by demonstrating their capacity for the work. It is a matter of finding the right balance. By striving for professional recognition, the family peer supporter runs the risk of becoming too closely aligned with the professional. Yet by being too distanced and critical of the professional, he or she runs another risk. Being too sharp a thorn in the team's side when advocating the family viewpoint can restrict, even block communication with the healthcare professionals. The family peer supporter should know the professional jargon well enough to give the family members a fair picture. But he or she should not be so familiar with the jargon that s/he uses it him/herself. As a member of the team, it is his/her task to actually remind healthcare professionals of the jargon they use, and to get them to speak in plain language to the patient's family.

Some family peer supporters, who prefer to keep their collaboration with healthcare professionals to a minimum, operate at a greater distance as a result of their own bad experiences. At some point in the past, they will have received little in the way of support when their family member was admitted to a psychiatric ward. For some, those bad experiences are what prompted them to become peer supporters in the first place. They now aim to secure the very thing they never received from healthcare professionals, and that is concern for and collaboration with the family. For this reason, they are less inclined to work closely with healthcare professionals and feel more useful as a thorn in the side. They are less inclined to come across as professional. And they see their work as parallel to that of the healthcare professional.

Of interest here is that family peer supporters are more often referred to families when they work with professionals as part of a team. The relationship of trust they have with their team colleagues and healthcare professionals is evidently vital when it comes to working with multiple families.

To my mind, it is important for a family peer supporter to have a good understanding of his role, both in his work with families and his contact with fellow healthcare professionals. Family peer supporters discuss these issues. They compare methods, such as distancing or close cooperation with the professionals, and assess their advantages and disadvantages. A discussion of these differences may allow them to develop a broader palette of mediations. It also allows them to explore a broader palette of relationships with healthcare professionals, and makes them able to choose the right mediation for the situation or the most appropriate stance opposite, alongside or in tandem with the healthcare professional. It seems to me that where collaborations with healthcare professionals are concerned, the visions of family peer supporters and fellow healthcare professionals should be very closely aligned when dealing with one and the same family. Family peer supporters should not be deployed simply if the healthcare professional is unable to establish contact with the family, or the family is perceived as an inconvenience, or even a nuisance, to the healthcare professional. If family peer supporters are only given the scope to operate when the professional has reached a dead end, the relationship of equality between the healthcare professional and the family peer supporter is at risk. It would make it seem that a family peer supporter can or should only operate in extreme circumstances, when all else has failed. This line of reasoning fails to appreciate the family peer supporter's role.

For some of the ward's patients, the process of trying to contact family ends in grief, because the contact appears irreparable. This is often the case for patients who ask family members to acknowledge the neglect or abuse they suffered. In the first place, the search for contact is often a search for acknowledgement of the abuse itself, by the offending family members. In this sense, the recovery work we do with families is a process through which the ending, or should I say provisional ending, is unpredictable, and in which it is more about being there through the process than about achieving the goal: the restoration of family relations.

Other family members that we cannot reach are those who have died. It is also important, of course, that we give them the space they deserve in the stories of the people we support. I have vivid memories, for example of a search undertaken by one person, who I counselled in relation to processing her father's death. He had died by suicide without leaving a note. He was a great support to her; so much so that she is certain her life would be completely different if he was still alive. Her journey is one of reconciling her love and loss of him with her sadness and anger at him for abandoning her by taking his own life. We set up a communication of a kind with her father in her own mind, through death, to try to bring her peace. Would she be able to understand him and accept what he did?

3.7 The Patient Perspective and Space

In his essay *Imperial Bedroom*, Jonathan Franzen talks about public spaces as places which shut out anything strictly private. He uses the museum as an example of such a place. People look around and can be seen by others, without sharing anything personal. There is a code governing the way you behave in these places.

> How sweet the promenading, the seeing and being seen. Everybody needs a promenade sometimes—a place to go when you want to announce to the world (not the little world of friends and family but the big world, the real world) that you have a new suit, or are in love, or suddenly realize that you stand a full inch taller when you don't hunch your shoulders.
>
> (Franzen, 1998, p. 50)

The public realm is a place where you want to reveal something of yourself without anyone knowing who you are, where you want to look at your best, show the pride you take in yourself. A long stay in a psychiatric hospital can threaten the very existence of this space. An essential part of who you are can be lost when you stay in a psychiatric hospital, by virtue of the fact that you are there. Your mere presence defines you as a patient. Anyone who comes for a long stay sees the sense of abject failure and isolation reflected in the others there. On a psychiatric hospital ward that public space has been swallowed by privacy.

81

Public space, the promenade, has ceased to exist there. The Italians have an even better word for the promenade: *la passeggiata*. The custom is to stroll around the old town, usually on a Sunday, to see and meet others, but it is just as important to be seen. They dress up specially. The elderly sit on benches and watch it all unfold. I have noticed that some people, after being on the ward for a long time, begin to let themselves go, stop caring about their appearance. I think this might have something to do with the loss of public space. When being 'a patient' is what everyone has in common, promenading, or showing yourself off and being seen, no longer happens. A psychiatric institution is not a place where you want to be seen. In the run-up to the New Year's Eve dinner, attended by neighbourhood residents, it always strikes me how, hours in advance, everyone gets ready, dresses up, to show themselves at their best. Obviously, even when in for a long stay, people are very conscious of the behavioural code in public spaces, the code of the promenade, and can take a great deal of pleasure in it. As well as connecting and coming into contact with others, it is important to belong to that public space and participate in it.

It has been the aim, since the psychiatric institution came into being, to remove people from the public realm. Pinel and Tuke saw isolation as a component of 'le traitement moral', and therefore as a means to a cure. In these institutions everything was based on, revolved around, a cure for the mentally ill patient. People were taken out of the public realm with a view to making them better again. They were taken to a place where they would have to learn to control themselves, and everything about that new environment told them that they were a patient (Hovius, 2013, p. 65). Not that long ago psychiatric hospitals were dinosaur institutions, with separate wards for men and women (the wards were not mixed until the 1980s). They had their own bakery, launderette, garden, woods, sports hall and swimming pool, a house for the psychiatrist, a staff canteen, a hairdresser's, a mortuary, a convenience store and, very importantly, a chapel. There was no need to leave the institution; everything was catered for. This meant that every conceivable, everyday activity, such as taking care of your hygiene, doing the shopping, going for a walk, was framed in a patient-staff context. The shopkeeper, a paid member of staff and non-patient, knew who was a patient and who was staff. Only very few members of staff would shop there in any case. The people who used the institution's facilities were patients, and the people who ran the facilities were paid workers. When people were admitted to the institution they lost their identity as a mother, father, man, woman... The profession you had once practised, the hobbies you once had, even your very past was engulfed by that sole identity, of which you were not proud, that sole identity of patient, that stripped you of your uniqueness as a person. In the end, with the loss of public space came the denial of your humanity. The diagnosis was all that remained. When you have been in a psychiatric institution for a long time you stop going to places where you can be seen and see others without being thought of as sick. You spend your life in a 'sick' community and may become unable to view yourself in any other way.

Spend years in an institution and you spend years, literally, being observed and viewed, always through the lens of the illness and diagnosis. You end up seeing yourself through the eyes of the healthcare professional, as a person who is in need of care and can no longer survive without it. This diagnostic mindset only reinforces your helplessness. With no hope of a life outside the psychiatric system, comes a downward spiral into despondency and a permanent distancing from self-responsibility. Many of the symptoms that complicate the patient-staff relationship are to do with this attitude of dependence. They reveal an inner but unrecognised struggle for more independence, which, the longer a stay progresses, produces a greater fear of that independence. In other words, the psychiatric institution was and is a totalitarian space, which reduces a group of people to a single identity, that of the sick person.

The toilet code in public spaces specifies one space for ladies and another for gents. On a psychiatric ward, they draw the line between staff and patients. Toilets for staff and toilets for patients. The right to a separate toilet is a matter set out in the employment contract. The frequent toilet-hygiene discussions will be altogether different, I would think, when toilets are shared with the staff. But it looks like this discussion will not be had, fortunately, as patients will have toilets in their own rooms in future. Marianne Farkas refers to the practice of maintaining separate toilets for staff and patients as 'bathroom-apartheid' (Marianne Farkas workshop entitled 'Het einde van het beschut wonen?' [The End of Sheltered Accommodation], organised by the non-profit Hand in Hand on 8 November 2016).

Anyone who has ever worked in a psychiatric institution will have seen it: the aquarium, or fish bowl. I am referring to the glass-walled nurses' station. They were originally designed as observation posts, from which, ideally, people could monitor the maximum number of corridors at once. Oversight and control, the symbols of power. There are many similarities between the institutions. All have nurses' stations. These are the places to which health-care professionals withdraw for briefings and consultations. Places that can be closed to patients. When the door is open, it is where patients often come for a chat. The chances of finding a nurse there are remarkably high.

The nurse sometimes uses this open space as a drop-in area, where people can wander freely in and out. Some patients come all the time, which makes others think that it is always busy and not the best place to get a nurse's attention. With all the comings and goings at these places, some healthcare professionals have a habit of switching their attention to the person who entered last, and away from the person who was there already. Often, several patients come in at once. Everyone talks at cross purposes. This breaks the conversations up, fragments them. The nurse that sees people in this central space gives attention from a spatial-organisation perspective. You have a real conversation with someone by finding a secluded spot and seeing to it that you are not disturbed. This cannot always be arranged if you are on duty alone and responsible for the ward. Every nurses' station has a computer on the table, with a monitor facing away, so that patients cannot read it when they enter. Privacy is paramount. One nurse behind the screen, almost as standard. These screens, linked to colleagues' computers, are the new observation windows through which information from colleagues now streams. Keeping up to date with what your colleagues see and do is an important way to keep a check on the latest arrangements for your patient. Most of the time the patient is unaware of what is written about him/her. This is the carers' domain. He/she can ask to see the file, but it does not happen often. It would be nice, for a change, to record observations with the patient's help. He/she would have to recognise the things reported about him/her. They would have to be insights designed to help him/her along the path s/he has chosen. Observations are recorded in other branches of medicine. Good observations give a better picture of the course of the disease and provide the basis for better treatment. In a general hospital, the most important observations are understood: temperature, blood pressure... But in a psychiatric hospital staff members often wonder what behaviour or statement to record in the notes. Is every observation worth recording? General hospitals do not record the visitors or the length of the visit. But psychiatric hospitals often do. It may useful, but then again it may not be. Is it important to record who gets on well with who, or to make assumptions about whether or not, for example, patients are having a relationship? Where does observation end and gossip begin? What is observation and what is interpretation? Is the behaviour we observe really as strange as we think? Does observed behaviour really have to be labelled as sick? And what information should or should not be shared with other healthcare professionals to allow us to continue our work with the client? Psychiatric observations take no account whatsoever of the place where they are made: the institution. If there is anything to be observed, it is mostly how a person behaves and feels when admitted to the institute, not how they behave outside. The observations are then interpreted, and, in the worst case, they confirm what the observers already suspect, i.e. that the subject belongs in the institution. Symptoms are then assembled into syndromes and linked to diagnoses. This creates a system of observation and categorisation in which the subjects cannot be anything other than patients, the very people who are meant to be there. Listen to these people, however, and you will hear stories of isolation, exclusion and stigmatisation. Many of these stories bear witness to the very consequences of having stayed in this sort of institution. For more reliable observations it is important to accompany patients to other places. As I have said, *en route* in the car, or on the bus, I have often seen and heard far more than I ever did while the patient was staying on the ward. People have really surprised me by being brilliant at finding their way around, for example, or by being far more socially adept than they appear on the ward. Others, who were dominant and quite blunt in their interactions with other patients, have turned out to be painfully shy with outsiders. In both cases, these observations led to the prognosis that they could handle themselves much better outside the ward than was initially thought. In the latter case, we got the idea that we just had to go out a lot more with this man to improve his social skills and help him overcome his fears.

> When I am in crisis, I don't stop to think where I am going, and then things usually turn out badly. I'll walk into a café and start drinking until I get aggressive. When I feel good I hardly dare put a foot outside the ward, because I'm afraid that I might get lost.

We do not get this statement until we have been out with him and seen how anxious he is on those occasions. The observation leads to a searching talk about himself. Due to the many crises, we see him in his worst light outside the institution and associate going out with crisis. By having more outings in non-crisis moments, he can exercise more control over his life and his future, and break free of his troubling dependence on the institution and his carers.

Nurses' stations are perfect to close off to patients and hold briefings and team meetings. They mark the boundary between patients and staff. In some places, staff still dress in white coats and sit at separate tables for coffee breaks and meals. The message here would seem to be one of difference and distance between staff and patients. Elements that signal a marked distinction between 'us' and 'them'.

In the days of 'moral treatment', it was believed that a building's structure could have a curative effect (Levin, 2005). Everything was seen in terms of therapy and treatment. This included the wrought iron and the structure of the corridors. Everything was arranged in an orderly manner in the belief that an uncluttered environment would lead to an uncluttered mind. This belief appears to have been abandoned. At present the hospital is associated with two functions: firstly, the provision of care and/or treatment, and, secondly, the provision of hotel services, such as food and beds. From the beginnings of 'moral treatment' until recently the hotel and treatment functions were understood as closely linked, and in this sense the term hotel function is fairly recent. Whereas at one time it was believed that the building itself could be restorative, we tend now to focus on where the building and ward environment might be a hindrance to a patient's self-management. We assess whether the hotel function on a ward might actually inhibit recovery. Lived experience expert, Hans Meganck:

> (free translation) At the ward where I was staying there were people in acute crisis as well as people who had been in treatment for

months. It didn't seem obvious to me. What I needed for my depression was peace and quiet mostly, which I couldn't get at all where I was staying. I was bothered by the constant stimuli: people mingling, mobile phones ringing all the time, the radio on all day. All in a fairly small living space. For real peace I had to go to my room, if my roommate would allow me any.

(Van Speybroeck, 2015)

'Having a rest' is still often cited as a reason for admission. The belief still exists that a stay on a ward can give a person rest by removing them from their everyday, debilitating environment. In isolation, away from family and friends, as a form of therapy. A similar argument is sometimes used to transfer someone from the open ward to the locked ward. It is thought that locking a person away will give the others more rest. Faced with this argument we may wonder who it is that needs the rest: in all likelihood the people closest to the patient, who are overtaxed, or the staff and other patients on the open ward, who can no longer cope with the restless patient. There is no shame in admitting that the behaviours of some patients can be exhausting. Recognising this and having the courage to discuss it with the patient is much more honest than claiming they need rest and should be taken away. Open and honest communication on this issue will give the patient an opportunity to tone down or change their behaviour, and so make life a little easier on the ward again. And a talk may be the very thing to provide alternatives that work for both parties.

Getting rest can be an important issue, but the psychiatric institution may not be the most appropriate setting for the hotel function. More and more ideas are being put forward to develop settings where people could actually get some rest, such as respite care homes. These places are outside the psychiatric ward. Respite care is a temporary, short-term stay in a care home, designed to support both you as the caregiver and the person you're caring for. If you're a caregiver, respite care lets you take a break or enables you to take time out to get things done. Places like these can be found in the UK. In the Netherlands, they are sometimes run by peer supporters. They give people the opportunity for a breather in a truly restful environment before returning to the domestic situation. They can also prevent an ineffective stay in a psychiatric institution. Greater variation in the hotel function is certainly advisable as a way to find peace and contemplate life. In the Netherlands, there are hotels who also provide some rooms for clients who want to take a break. A buddy is available during the stay, along with different combinations of treatment or support. They are great places to slow the pace, far from the bustle. People may feel more like a person, not a patient, as there are no therapies. But many places do still offer the hotel function alongside therapies. Keeping your room tidy and preparing your own meals are regarded as essentials, and they are mandatory. Here, people with mental ill health are still often seen by some caregivers as overly passive and in need of activation. I would say that this line of reasoning is open to criticism. Ending up in a psychiatric institution is enough to depress anyone, which is why people may become inactive. They can feel depressed because they have ended up on this railway siding. And sticking with a therapy is no guarantee that they will continue the activity after discharge. Transferring the activities outside the institution is questionable for many reasons. Activities cannot be automatically transferred from one place to another. In the Netherlands, this rationale is criticised as 'dry swimming': doing swimming strokes on the floor is no way to learn how to swim. To do that, you have to be in the water.

> Chris, who has cooked for years in an inpatient setting stops cooking at home because it hardly seems worth only cooking for one. I pay him a visit, as his case manager, at which point he decides to cook again, because he likes the idea of making us both a meal. The place and circumstances of a person's stay have a massive effect on their level of activity.
>
> Mario is admitted to the ward. At a halfway house he has been taken through the preparations for living in sheltered accommodation. The support workers there tell us that Mario is obviously not ready for sheltered housing, due to repeated relapses into substance abuse. The probation service backs this recommendation. They want to send Mario on a lengthy drug-use programme. The assignment nurse wants Mario to get a place in sheltered housing within a week of joining our ward, as he has been on the list for a very long time. Mario is desperately keen to go. He is sick and tired of long-stay admissions. With 'housing first' in mind, our team recommends that we give this a try. We suggest that Mario come to us for day-patient therapy, so that we can keep an eye on his development in the new housing situation. This brings us into a network that emphasises coaching at home. After three years, Mario is still in sheltered housing. In all that time he has not relapsed. Later Mario tells us that drug abuse was rife among the residents of the halfway house where he was being prepared for sheltered housing. The halfway house was actually a dedicated facility for substance abusers. He was tempted to use drugs every time the others did. There are no users where Mario lives now, which is why he feels good. 'Just let me live somewhere that isn't full of drug users,' he said. The simple solution is to listen to him; contrast that with a system in which healthcare professionals believe they can teach courses in independent living, and that the results are transferable to another place. Support and training 'on the ground' seem to be so much more effective, provided they are given in the right place.

It seems important to me, in mental healthcare, that the psychiatric institution should be a part of the network around the patient, but not be at its centre. The patient should be at the centre. It is s/he who is in control. The main objective of the ward in a psychiatric institution is to make way for the social services, especially those that provide care in the home. Known information on the patient is disclosed, with the patient's consent, to the providers of home support. The real work begins when the patient leaves the institution. From the institutional perspective this is 'aftercare'. From the client perspective, aftercare is actual care.

If the ward, with all its hotel functions, activities, therapies, and so on, is no longer the central hub within which treatment brings about the desired change in the patient, what is the purpose of an admission at the present time?

Gideon Boie, architect and philosopher:

> (free translation) What can be the central reference on a ward? Perhaps it should be the room, like a hotel room, where the patient can organise his life temporarily. A hotel is also conceived through its relationship to external factors, because a hotel is located somewhere in the area and is organised around that environment.
>
> (Van Speybroeck, 2015, p. 10)

Our main interest on our ward is to help the patient relate to his or her future environment. Therefore we see the ward as a base, and an entirely provisional base, because people always run the risk of being less able to take control of their lives when they stay for a long time. The care team on the ward is very outreaching to the patient in his future environment.

An active, enterprising care worker who conveys a message of hope and confidence to a patient in his/her care is largely interested in the patient's personal story and relationships with immediate friends, family and other significant parties, and it does not matter whether these people are alive or dead. From this perspective the ward experience is not the core of the work, and the ward itself is not the hub from which meetings are arranged.

If there is a hub in the ward, then, as in any hotel, it is the patient's room. Here, the word 'hotel' implies that staff are there to serve the guest, and, through coaching in his or her hub, i.e. room, to give him/her the support needed to reintegrate and find a life of quality and meaning.

If maximum self-management is important, you have to emphasise made-to-measure service, as well as the highly individual pathway taken by every patient. We offer variation in the ward's accommodation. Hence the availability of short-stay beds, so that people can return to us if they briefly need the safety of interaction with familiar healthcare professionals on the ward, without too many questions or intake formalities.

We make sure that a variety of hotel and coaching combinations is available, and we do this by keeping the two entirely separate for the purpose of delivering made-to-measure services. If we notice that someone on the ward is still in need of treatment, we have the option of arranging this at another unit, because that unit is more specialised and has greater expertise in the area concerned. We make an arrangement with the treatment unit to read-mit the patient to us afterwards, so they can continue the process of reso-cialising and finding work and accommodation. Interviews are sometimes arranged with a psychologist outside the institution while the patient is still on the ward, to guarantee continuity of care when the patient leaves. On the other hand, a patient who is about to be discharged can continue to see the ward psychologist for a time as part of the aftercare service.

3.8 Patient Perspective and Safety

One of the key words on a psychiatric ward is safety. In her workshop enti-tled 'The End of Sheltered Accommodation?' (Ghent, 8 November 2016) Marianne Farkas spoke about provider-centred services, which we have described above as aspects of the organisation. These are mostly based on control, risk and fear, whereas recovery-centred services are based on the patients' strength, choices, hopes and dreams and on providing patients with more opportunities for a meaningful life.

The difference in approach can produce entirely different solutions to the same problem. Patient-centred measures are made to measure for the per-son; organisation-centred measures are always standard by definition, and therefore never custom-made. This is something to be borne in mind.

Organisations must have safety measures, this is a fact. Rules are needed, for everyone's safety, when people (healthcare professionals and patients) live together in numbers. But these rules can be very restrictive for the patients who stay there. The challenge, as we see it, is to stay focused on safety, but to keep looking for ways to achieve it without harming the patient. Although coercive measures are effective in maintaining safety on the ward, they can be highly traumatising for anyone who experiences them.

Force and pressure are no longer considered therapeutic, in our team we see it as a necessary evil. In Belgium, alternatives such as 'Soteria' and 'Open Dialogue' crop up here and there. At this stage they seem fairly labour-intensive, and are not yet common practice. While on the FACT Team I notice that on home visits healthcare professionals will stay present with distressed or aggressive people for much longer than they do on the ward. The mere existence of a bigger arsenal of safety measures (placement on the locked ward, more staff on locked wards, isolation cells...) increases the chances of these measures being used. Apparently, higher levels of staff responsibility on the ward, to maintain safety, make the care team more likely to resort to force and pressure through more drastic measures.

A minor is involuntarily admitted to a youth ward because he has stopped going to school. A hotel function, a stay where he does not wish to be, is imposed along with the treatment. While there, he is tested and found to have a slight learning difficulty. He is traumatised, firstly by the admission, but more so by the test results. No one considers the stress induced by the situation at the time of testing, or that Dutch is not his native language. As an adult, years after this involuntary admission, he rarely leaves the house. It takes him a long time to trust the healthcare professionals who visit him at home. The counselling at home, the conversations, are about processing the trauma he experienced in a psychiatric unit. A trauma which he is unable to overcome until he completes his professional training. Only then can he believe that he does not have a mental disability. Only then is he truly convinced of his ability, and can he put that dreadful experience, from years ago, behind him. It is not unusual for a healthcare professional to need to provide therapy for the traumas a person has suffered in the psychiatric system.

There are ways to make the locked ward less traumatic for the patient. In the high intensive care-model, a 'high-care-function' and an 'intensive-care function' are combined. Initially, patients are admitted on the High Care section (HC). In case stress, anxiety and agitation rise, or when aggression is imminent, one-to-one care can be given at the HC, or depending on the severity and nature of the crisis patients can go (accompanied by a nurse of the HC), to the Intensive Care Unit (ICU). Under HIC or High Intensive Care, which has been around in the Netherlands for a number of years, friends and relatives are allowed to stay in the patient's room overnight during a stay on a locked ward. Working with patients and their families involves a willingness to share your own territory, the ward, by openly acknowledging the expertise of patients and family members. It is the only way to make the ward more like a public space and less authoritarian. For the time being, it seems that sharing territory on the ward with a patient's friends, family or other important people, is not yet acceptable in most psychiatric institutions around the world.

For the sake of safety, patients suffer a huge loss of privacy in the institution. There are rules to be followed by the night staff on the ward. One of the duties is to open the door several times a night to check that a patient is sleeping and that everything is okay.

(free translation) The night time check on my first crisis admission threw me into total panic... I hadn't been told about it, and I imagined the perpetrator in my room... it never got any better... the night staff, though well intentioned, were always an absolute threat during my crisis admissions.... A second experience: during my long admission my girlfriend threw herself under a train. I withdrew to my bed, in total shock... Every half hour somebody came 'to look at me' = to see if was still alive.... nobody asked me anything, started a conversation.... They came to look...' (Wilma Boevink, conversation with me on Facebook).

If checks by night staff are comforting, it is because staff make time for a chat if the patient is awake. Being observed and checked doesn't really give a sense of security, but talking does. Some measures, introduced through concern or for reasons of safety, may create a sense of insecurity if the human aspect is ignored.

The patients cannot open the windows in their rooms. Again, this is to do with safety. It can be quite unpleasant in the summertime. It is impossible for patients to ventilate their rooms. And that can be hard on someone who is particular about hygiene.

Like general hospitals, psychiatric hospitals operate strict rules of hygiene: animals are not allowed in the institution, meals can't be stored in the fridges... These rules create a sterile environment, literally and figuratively. Safety combined with an organisation-centred-care mindset ('We know what is good for you because we've thought long and hard about it') often leads to rules that serve the largest common denominator or average patient, when no such thing exists. These rules have a total disregard for the individual. By matching the sequence of what we say and do with the wishes of the patient, thoughts on the issue of safety can be tailored to the individual.

An admission to a psychiatric institution is an extremely complex event. Patients are forced to question their own autonomy, and this is a difficult step, especially if they were unable to rely on other significant people in their childhood. The patient may lack a basic sense of security, so even the slightest surrender of control to another person seems to carry a heavy risk. The ward of a psychiatric institution may seem like the right place to look for security, but severely traumatised people sense any relinquishment of control as deeply dangerous, and therefore frightening and stressful. Allowing someone to take care of you still carries a fear of abuse. The fact that your hosts own the building, and can put you on the street if they want to, only adds to the stress. The stress is there to see, but the patient cannot speak of it without revealing his or her vulnerability. Tensions can reach breaking point, and very close work with the patient is needed to keep this temporary arrangement liveable. There is a danger that s/he might become a revolving-door patient, moving from one institution to another, endlessly seeking help without ever relinquishing control.

> Brian has been admitted, and he wants help. He is not asking for it. He is demanding it. But the help we give is always inadequate, always insufficient. He says that we don't take good enough care of him. We listen hard, but still he is dissatisfied. To accept help is to tolerate dependence. He will not tolerate it, because he does not trust the healthcare workers, not any more. He was mistreated as a child. He looks for security in us, wants to be helped, but fears that we might abuse our power too. He will not, cannot, allow himself to

be vulnerable, so he makes demands and orders us to care for him. He says he can do a better job himself, and that he will prove it. He wants to assume our work with the other patients. He knows them better than we do. Here, the desire for security and the need for absolute independence are entwined in an extraordinary way. An untenable situation. He finds accommodation. By giving him his independence we rid ourselves of the need to be endlessly concerned with the conflicts that erupt around him on the ward. He can make a new request for support without feeling helpless, without fear that we will take advantage of that helplessness. Living independently, he no longer finds himself in an untenable position with us.

The security of a ward can be a trap that is difficult to escape. 'A long admission can affect your ability to reassure yourself', says expert by experience Sonja Visser, on a visit to our ward in 2016. Staying in institutions for a long time creates a special dynamic, and it affects everyone who ends up in this position. Being homeless and on the ward of a psychiatric unit creates a dynamic that affects every citizen, irrespective of diagnosis. This dynamic places security and independence in a kind of diametric opposition.

Helga packs her bags. She hadn't realised how much stuff she has gathered over the years of admissions. A smile tinged with sadness. The admission gave her security. We see her associate with the strongest on the ward and criticise the weakest. They won't engage with therapy, won't do the washing up... While the ward gives her security, we see that it is an unpleasant place for her to be, because in her eyes the patients don't try their best. She is wrapped up in the minutiae of ward life. She feels a huge responsibility for the ward. It takes up almost all of her energy. We tell her that she has outgrown the ward, that she is entitled to a nicer environment, and that it really does exist outside the ward. But she gets anxious at the thought of leaving. Fear of leaving the security of the ward, fear of failure: the price she has to pay for more independence, a nicer place, a place of her own to furnish. We tell her that this is the point she has grown to in the last two years: a home, a place of her own, to furnish herself, where the only people around are the people of her choosing. She asks if we are sending her away. She is so used to being sent away. So used to rejection. I smile and tell her that she is always very welcome on the ward. She will come for day therapy. We will still see each other a lot and, of course, we will talk a lot, about her unprocessed experiences, her childhood traumas. There is still much to be done. The treatment will continue, only she won't have to stay on the ward. Leaving this place, a place of security for her, is not being sent away. It is letting go. Beginning a new phase of her life, getting stronger, becoming less dependent. It doesn't mean her problems have all been solved. We run over her crisis plan, her favourite music when she feels bad, her emergency medication, and now the idea that she can visit or call us at any time of day. The nurses and therapists she knows so well are still available. And yes, she can call the night staff, if she wants to. She counts down the days and a greater freedom and independence open before her like untold possibilities. And very briefly I feel like a father watching a child fly the nest.

3.9 Hope

Besides security and independence the dynamic of a stay on a ward involves a third factor, and that is hope. The longer you remain in a problematic situation, the more likely you are to lose hope of ever escaping it. Hope is the very thing you need in order to find the strength for change. One sign of a good healthcare professional is the ability in the first place to rekindle a patient's hope for a better future. If a patient has had frequent and long admissions, s/he can only do this by being and staying present, especially when things go wrong.

A passive and overly reassuring attitude on the part of a healthcare professional, in a world that piles one misery on top of another, can be tremendously damaging for inpatients. It can make patients lose their zest for life. An inviting attitude, and giving hope as well as being present, can give people the courage to get going again and reclaim their place in society.

In *De nacht van Nederland* Marius Nuy (2001, p. 24) talks about homeless people who have the ability to reflect on themselves and their own situation and have not suffered childhood trauma. They are soon recognised by healthcare professionals in the homeless circuit as people who do not belong on the street. Their self-reflection and vitality give them the tools to escape a situation which is essentially alien to them. They usually manage it under their own steam. Healthcare professionals seem to identify the overwhelming majority of homeless people as a specific group, and take the attitude that a circuit of this kind is the right place for them. A very traumatic childhood has left some form of homelessness imprinted on their mind. Some homeless people are unable to reflect on themselves. For instance because of a slight mental disability. That is another element that robs them of the strength to escape this degrading situation. But healthcare professional should stop seeing them as people who have ended up where they belong, i.e. homeless.

'On this point the demands on care providers are much greater than is often thought. In the care setting it is not about a bed and a bowl of soup, those are given, but helping to find the "size that fits" – which is undiscoverable for many homeless people – and together seeing which context offers the best opportunities for a future. After all, nobody should have to rely exclusively on their own devices; in care, particularly, everyone can have faith in serious, respectful and pragmatic assistance, with plenty of "lifelines" on offer. Because anyone who does not have the natural ability to self reflect, must "otherwise" be helped in more specific ways (...) the tragedy is that it is sometimes believed that many "simply belong here" and appear to be "at home". It is as if they (almost) all look the same, and separate identities no longer matter. This is the antithesis of authenticity. We cannot and should not stop investigating an individual's prospects, and taking advantage of opportunities, even if they initially look slim, although it can be "a slow process.

(Nuy, 2001, p. 24)

The professional distance, the cold and impersonal treatment, the absurd application and interpretation of rules and protocols is demeaning and harmful, but, beyond that, it robs people of hope for an upturn in their situation. The actual dynamics of an admission bring dangers, and we should be aware of this. It is important for all that work in an institution to understand the attractive force, the gravity of a totalitarian institution like psychiatry. The paradox seems to be that on entering the psychiatric system, people need to have the strength to escape it. Healthcare professionals in psychiatric institutions must keep trying to create and maintain a movement and dynamic that puts patient self-management first, without abandoning or neglecting the person in the process. It is necessary to give hope for a future outside the institution and to work very actively towards that.

The good healthcare professional discovers and realises that hope can lie concealed behind a patient's anger and rage, and that it is best for him/her to recognise this anger and rage as a strength, even if the rage is initially directed at the healthcare professional or the institution s/he represents. On the ward we recognise this obstinacy, this resistance, as a force that drives people and inspires them to action, gets them thinking beyond a life on the ward. This is the very force (wanting to escape detention and residence in the psychiatric system, fighting to have your children nearer to you, fighting for a better society) that drives people to survive. The first thing you do as a healthcare professional is view this resistance or anger as a source of energy to enable change; the idea is to embrace the energy as an ally in the battle to reclaim hope for change. Providing fertile ground for something new to grow from the energy behind the anger is good care practice.

Sheila has just been admitted to the ward. She walks into the nurses' station, protesting loudly. We are doing it all wrong. By 'we' she means the healthcare professionals, the staff and, therefore, the representatives of the psychiatric system. She wants to be heard, because she has a better idea of how it should be done. Her assigned nurse takes the time to listen. The woman talks about her mission to save the world. Her very specific mission is to rescue every child in need. To fulfil it, she is in contact with a famous American rapper. She has to carry out her programme, and she has to do it through his songs. She listens to his music all the time, because the lyrics contain a message for her. Her daughter was taken from her, because she was no longer able, through her addiction, to look after her. She has not visited her daughter, who is now in a care home, for some time. Recently, a failed consultation appointment served only to increase the distance between her and her daughter's support workers. We concentrate on the sorrow she feels at losing her daughter. We situate her anger in this context. We investigate the possibility of improving communication between her and her daughter, and we help her get in touch with the authorities and care workers entrusted with her daughter's support. Her daughter's well-being is also a matter of great importance to us. She is talking to our ward psychologist. They come to an arrangement over medication. Here too, she is in control. We see to it that she can stay in touch with the healthcare professionals she knows and trusts. We encourage this, and we also stay in touch with them. We speak to her parents and see to it that the connection is rebuilt. And so we build a network. After a few months of working together she says that she has something to tell me, and that she is very ashamed of it. She says that for a long time she believed that she was in contact with a rapper, that he was talking to her and that she and he were on a mission to make the world a better place. She tells me that they are no longer in touch. She asks me, very cautiously, if I think she is mad. I tell her that for a while she needed the rapper's help, because she couldn't cope with it all alone, and that now she is stronger she doesn't need his help. That those experiences, so strange to her now, were necessary to her survival at the time. She is glad to hear that I think she is a madwoman and understands the logic of being able to move ahead by herself now. In further conversations she talks about music and its importance to her, and she says she misses the rapper. She says she spends more time in reality, but that it often feels cold and eerie because she has to face it more alone now. She misses him, and the harshness of life can get to her at times, but she wants to keep going. On the drive home from a meeting with her daughter's network she tells me about the importance of her grandmother, who has since passed away. She had a really strong bond with her. Her grandmother would regularly say, 'sing a song if you feel sad and everything will get better'. We lay out the pieces of the puzzle: a much-loved grandmother who advised her to seek solace in music in difficult times, her immense sorrow and feeling of powerlessness at losing her daughter and her contact with a rapper, a musician, through which she believed that she could make the world a better place, especially for children. In ensuing conversations it emerges, through her feelings of missing the rapper, that she misses her grandmother. The two are connected by music. More memories follow and her past, present and future appear to be moving in line. The psychotic experiences make sense and have meaning. The original anger, which came with the task of world saviour, is now far behind us, but it was this anger that enabled connection, and this anger that sparked her recovery. Hearing and seeing her anger as a response to an injustice done to her was the starting point in the therapeutic relationship.

It is vital to have the energy needed to live. Sometimes this vital energy comes out as rage and unruliness. It should not be our goal to transform the unruliness to peace and calm, or resignation to a stay with no prospect of a future beyond the institution, because this is the very thing that stills the dynamic. The anger often marks the necessary direction of change in the world beyond the institution, and the means of achieving that change is often connection and collaboration. In terms of effort and social engagement, then, much is expected of the healthcare professional. However, the peace and calm with which we often act and operate in a psychiatric institute should never give way to resignation, for resignation places the interests of the patient at risk. A hands-on, active input, often literally walking a path, and the many phone calls and emails written with the person to significant people (family, previous healthcare professionals, coaches, home support workers, etc.) renews the connections and reinvigorates communication.

Some patients, who come across as angry or psychotic, risk communicating in a manner that stops people from listening to what they are saying. On the ward we try to channel this anger, so the content can be heard. A few of these ways to channel are rooted in our desire for a more humane psychiatry. We create our own socially engaged work groups, such as *Kiosk*. In this magazine created on the ward, we give people the opportunity to write about unjustice. It is part of our community outreach project. We create channels of our own to actually pave the way for change, in the psychiatric landscape and beyond. The patients play a very active part in our actions for a more humane psychiatry, and this gives their anger over injustice a socially acceptable outlet towards change. In the first place, we are companions.

We ask one extremely passionate patient, who often sides against us, if we can literally join forces, be companions. We raise the idea of joining forces when the effort serves a higher purpose: the fight against injustice. And if there is one injustice that the psychiatric patient knows all about, it is exclusion. Let the fight against this particular injustice be the very purpose of what we do through quartermaking. Another patient, who wants a better world and fights hard against injustice, speaks at a meeting of our Flemish Working Group on Quartermaking. She makes a notable call for more respect and collaboration and is given a round of applause for her contribution. It does her a power of good. For the first time in a long while her anger is greeted with approval. In the heart of the dogged warrior there is often hope, for without it he would give up the fight. The people who give up fighting are often the ones who have given up hope. Coaches give them hope for the future, as they can be companions and comrades in arms. Taking action to find or create your own space is often the only way to send the faltering dynamic of safety and independence in a new direction.

The example below, of 'housing first' covers all of the observations made above. We spoke about patient time rather than ward time, and we spoke about the very specific dynamic induced by a long stay on a ward. We spoke about the importance of being a 'hope provider' for the people you support.

Mary was referred to us from a treatment ward. And we were told by caregivers from this ward that she was 'a borderline case'. The diagnosis was very stigmatising. She has been homeless for several years and has no other option but to move from one institution to another. Many of these places have thrown her onto the street. The healthcare professionals there have said she is impossible to work with. She is quite withdrawn and disinterested in the therapies on the ward. She refuses to have any individual talks.

She is described as a person who demands all kinds of practical help: from collecting her clothes from the storage facility a few miles down the road, to taking her to see her mother. Her demands are endless. She refuses to speak of her past or about what matters to her. She won't participate in group conversations and frequently acts out. She gets verbally aggressive if her demands are not met, and there are conflicts with fellow patients, as a result of which she often ends up on the locked ward. Once there, the aggression continues until she is eventually restrained. The ward is advised stick to talking and not to entertain her demands for practical help. We have been told that she will try to play us. She is manipulative, they add. Nobody would escort her on a visit to her mother's. It has been years since she has seen her. They wanted to stick to talking, in other words. They didn't think she was ready for independent living. They wanted to hear her talk, to identify the factors that led to her homelessness. Their observation of the many difficulties on the ward confirm their opinion that she cannot live independently and reveal the areas in which her thinking and behaviour will have to change if she is to be considered for independent living. While she continues to exhibit problem behaviour on the ward, she is not ready to leave. Openings cannot be found with words, and so the healthcare professionals believe that she will never be able to live alone and will have to spend the rest of her life on a long-stay ward. The referral to that long-stay ward is on hold, as there are no places available. We happen to have room on our ward, and she is referred to us by chance. People seem almost apologetic for the referral.

When we remind her referrers of our vision, to return people to society by allowing them to live independently or in sheltered accommodation, they wish us the very best of luck and add that it will never work.

My first real contact with her on the active rehab ward is a conversation in the car on the way to her mother's. It is hard work, full of silences. Afterwards, I get the impression that the visit to her mother's hadn't really gone too well, but she makes out that everything was okay. Later, after a few more car journeys to take care of practicalities, we will begin to talk about the visit in more depth, as we do about her wishes, her past and her future. Taking action, getting out and about with her, doing things together, generates trust, and through this the most significant conversations will arise. But one thing truly strengthens the bond between her, myself and the other healthcare professionals, and that is our unconditional acceptance of her request for rented accommodation. The *housing first* principle rests on the idea that everyone is entitled to a home and that it needn't be conditional on treatment or coaching. Until now, the only place she has had is in a psychiatric hospital, as a patient. The healthcare professionals imagined that she would need treatment first and thereafter, step-by-step, through sheltered accommodation in a house with former patients, she could work towards independent living. We, on the rehabilitation ward, see her as a citizen entitled to a home as much as any other citizen. We take her request for independent living seriously and do not see her issues on the ward as a predictor of future difficulties with independent living. We support her unconditionally in her search for a home. She is offered a place through the social housing agency. At that very moment, I join the FACT Team and can continue to coach her at home. It works. She manages to live independently. After a year she decides that she is having a difficult time and asks for a brief admission to a treatment ward in another hospital. She is known to them after a previous stay, and they take a very deep breath before admitting her, because she had acted out almost constantly. To their surprise, however, she turns out to be a model patient on this occasion. Later, she talks about the difference herself. On the new admission she has a home to return to, so she has more control over her life. She won't be on the street if they discharge her. And, since we on the FACT Team will continue our unconditional support, she won't have to face it alone if she is discharged. If she feels that the treatment doesn't suit her needs, she is free to discharge herself without a problem.

The intolerable dependence that comes with being admitted while homeless had triggered a feeling of conflict in her that went back to the total helplessness she experienced as a victim of sexual abuse. Back then she was entirely at the mercy of a person who abused their power, the very person who was supposed to provide safety. Previous admissions had been complicated by the sheer inequality of the relationship, the powerlessness, the dependency on others for a roof over her head, and so the treatments had failed. To healthcare professionals and fellow patients on the ward she came across and untreatable and aggressive and regularly found herself on the locked ward, where they even resorted to restraining her. Her dependence and powerlessness were demonstrated to us in what was a destructive relationship for her and a frustrating one for us, a power game that was wanted by no one and in which we, as healthcare professionals, were in danger of being complicit. A different attitude, without the obvious power imbalance, was the only way out. We gave her support, and the hope of being in control of her life, by helping her find a home. With a home, she is in a position to make a genuine request for treatment.

Not being homeless when admitted to the psychiatric ward gives her a status on top of that of a 'patient': the status of citizen. The admission and having a place to stay are not one and the same. She already has a home, and this separation of the two statuses gives her the security she needs to commence treatment at the institution. When admitted, a homeless person may not separate the living function from the treatment function. The dynamic this introduces can undermine the treatment. The *housing first* principle makes treatment possible in the long term, if still needed. Today she is in a relationship, has lived with her boyfriend for several years, and has completed her training. We meet up occasionally for a coffee and a chat. We laugh about the healthcare professionals who gave up on her because she wouldn't talk.

The picture of recovery outlined in this chapter represents the first component of community-based care, in which we do not see clients as the bearers of a diagnosis, with add-on disabilities, but as citizens who have the right to a home, a job and the ability to do something meaningful with their time. People should not have to demonstrate a sufficient level of health before these rights come into play. The new definition of health or recovery is all about patients being able to exercise enough control over their lives. Housing is extremely important when it comes to giving a person more control. Treatment can then be organised in accordance with the housing situation. The healthcare professionals at the institution are the ones who ensure continuity of treatment, by either continuing it themselves if the patient finds a home, or transferring it to a network that includes healthcare professionals who provide home care.

New healthcare professionals build on the results that we have all achieved together on our ward. We decentralise our services by looking for reliable, new healthcare professionals in the region who practice, as we do, according to recovery-oriented principles. We remain a point of contact for these new healthcare professionals, and a place of rest for former patients, a place where trusted and known persons can be found to come to grips with new things. Above all, we see ourselves as a step-up to something different, outside the mental healthcare setting.

The second movement that ties in very closely with recovery is quarter-making. The citizens we come across on our psychiatric wards are people who are excluded, who stand in the margins, and, as healthcare professionals, we should make sure that something is done about that exclusion.

References

Andries Baart and Christa Carbo, *De zorgval. Analyse, kritiek en uitzicht*, Amsterdam, Thoeris, 2013.

W. Boevink, M. Prins, L. Elfers, J. Droës, M. Tiber and G. Wilrycx, Herstel ondersteunende zorg, een concept in ontwikkeling. *Tijdschrift voor Rehabilitatie*, 1, 42–54, 2009.

F.A.L. Campos, A.R. Pinto de Sousa, V.P da Costa Rodrigues, A.J. Pereira da Silva Marques, A.A. Monteiro da Rocha Dores, C.M. Liete Queiros, Peer support for people with mental illness. *Revista de Psiquiatria Clínica*, 41(2), 49–55, 2014.

Nick Cave, One more time with feeling (documentary director Andrew Dominik), 2016.

John Conolly, *An inquiry concerning the indications of insanity*, London, John Taylor, 1830.

P.A.E.G. Delespaul, *Terug naar af met de GGZ? Pleidooi voor een innovatieve en duurzame psychische hulpverlening*, Maastricht University. https://doi.org/10.26481/spe.20130411pd, 2013.

Thomas Detombe, Psychiaters over dwang en vrijheidsbeperking — achtergrond — Sociaal.Net, januari 2022.

Joke De Witte en Hans Van Dartel, dilemma, een cadeautje aannemen van een zorgvrager. *V & VN Magazine*, 2019.

P. Dierinck, We gaan de teamvergadering afschaffen — Column — Sociaal.Net juni, 2022.

D.B. Double, The history of anti-psychiatry: An essay review. *History of Psychiatry*, 13, 231–236, 2002.

J. Dröes and J. Van Weeghel, Perspectieven van psychiatrische rehabilitatie. *Maandblad Geestelijke Volksgezondheid*, 49(8), 795–810, 1994.

Familie als partner in de ggz, een praktische gids voor zorgverleners, Similes, 2012.

Marianne Farkas Workshop, Het einde van het beschut wonen? [The End of Sheltered Accommodation?], organised by the non-profit Hand in Hand on 8 November 2016.

John Foot, *The man who closed the asylums, Franco Basaglia and the revolution in Mental Health Care*, London and New York, VersoBooks, 2015.

Michel Foucault, *History of madness*, Abingdon, Oxon, Routledge, 2009.

Jonathan Franzen, Imperial bedroom. *The New Yorker*, October 5, 1998.

Brenda Froyen, *Psychotic mum: An inside story*, Gent, Borgerhoff & Lamberigts, 2019.

Gids naar een betere geestelijke gezondheidszorg, 2002. http://www.psy107.be/files/Vlaanderen.pdf.

J.M. Held, Expressing the inexpressible, Lyotard and the differend. *Journal of the British Society for Phenomenology*, 36(1), 76–89, 2005.

Liza Hopkins, Supporting the support network: The value of family peer work in Youth Mental Health Care. *Community Mental Health Journal*, 57(2), 926–936, 2021.

Ranne Hovius, *De eenzaamheid van de waanzin. Tweehonderd jaar psychiatrie in romans en verhalen*, Amsterdam, Nieuwezijds, 2013.

M.A.S. Huber, *Towards a new, dynamic concept of health: Its operationalisation and use in public health and healthcare and in evaluating health effects of food*, Maastricht, Maastricht University, 2014.

M.A.S. Huber, M. Van Vliet, M. Giezenberg, B. Winkens, Y. Heerkens, P.C. Dagnelie, J.A. Knottnerus, Towards a 'patient-centred' operationalisation of the new dynamic concept of health: A mixed methods study. *BMJ Open* 12, 6(1), e010091. doi: 10.1136/bmjopen-2015-010091, 2016.

Doortje Kal, *Kwartiermaken. Werken aan ruimte voor mensen met een psychiatrische achtergrond*, Amsterdam, Boom, 2001.

Marijke Kars, *Parenting and palliative care in paediatric oncology*, Utrecht, Julius Center for Health Science and Primary Care, UMC/UU, 2012.

R.D. Laing, *The divided self*, London, Penguin Modern Classics, 1965.

A. Levin, *Rational buildings designed to 'calm the disorderly mind'*, Washington D.C., American Psychiatric Association, 2005.

Hans Meganck, Stephan De Bruyne and Marjolein Deceulaer, *Depressief. Goede zorg voor kwetsbare mensen*, Tielt, Lannoo, 2014.

Loren R. Mosher, H. Voyce, D.C. Fort, *Soteria: Through madness to deliverance*, Xlibris Corporation, 2004.

Martha C. Nussbaum, *Frontiers of justice: Disability, nationality, species membership*, Cambridge MA, Harvard University Press, 2007.

Marius Nuy, *De nacht van Nederland*, Amsterdam, SWP, 2001.

D. Oaks, The evolution of the consumer movement. *Psychiatric Services*, 57(8), 1212, 2006.

Detlef Petry, *Uitbehandeld maar niet opgegeven. Het persoonlijke verhaal van een psychiater over zijn patiënten*, Amsterdam, Ambo, 2011.

Heather Plett, What it means to 'hold space' for people, plus eight tips on how to do it well, website http://heatherplett.com/2015/03/hold-space/.

ed. Nick Putman and Brian Martindale, *Open dialogue for psychosis*, Abingdon, Routledge, 2021.

Marita Törrönen, C. Munn-Giddings, L. Tarkiainen, *Reciprocal relationships and well-being*, Abingdon, Routledge, 2019.

Ann Van de Vloet, *Een nieuwe wind waait door Uilenspiegel*, Brussel, Spiegel, 2013–2014.

Jan Van Speybroeck, Dirk Armée, Gideon Boie, Mieke Craeymeersch, Jan Delvaux, Peter Dierinck, Hans Meganck and Fie Vandamme, Psychiatrisch ziekenhuis of all-in zorghotel, Over milieutherapie, maatwerk, stigma en droogzwemmen. *Tijdschrift psychiatrie en verpleging*, 91(4), 6–12, 2015.

4

CARE IN THE COMMUNITY

Quartermaking

4.1 Through Italy to Belgium and the Municipality

The statement below by Basaglia, refers to a movement that emphasises quartermaking.

'How can we not move from the excluded to the excluder?' (Basaglia in Foot, 2015, p. 180). In the late 1960s Franco Basaglia leaves Gorizia. He had intended to reform and close the psychiatric hospital there. But, in the wake of the internal reforms, making the institution less repressive, everything comes to a dead end. He is unable to work in the therapeutic community he created. A new team comes in to continue his work.

> The next day the new équipe attended their first general assembly. Realdon remembered 'an enormous room full of people, smoke, coughing, confused voices shouting. Her overall conclusion was that this reformed hospital had become a trap (...) She argued that one of the reasons that it was difficult to reduce the numbers in the hospital was the central role played by the patients inside the asylum itself. Outside they were nobody; inside they were part of a Basaglian therapeutic community. It was as if the perfection of the Basaglia system was preventing patients from taking responsibility for their lives. Like the Basaglians, Realdon felt that Gorizia had become a 'golden cage'.
>
> (Ibid., p. 318)

Also now empowering people inside the psychiatric hospital seems merely to make them feel important while inside. When they try to take their place in society, the sense of having any real significance vanishes. This makes them prefer, above all else, to stay in the institution. Only there are they of real significance.

Later, when describing his work in Trieste, Basaglia wrote:

> the opening up of the hospital and freedom of communication can only work if the external world participates as one part of the

DOI: 10.4324/9781003220015-5

relationship – freedom of communication will remain an artifice if we are unable to open up and keep a dialogue going between the internal and external worlds... It is necessary at this stage that the external world recognizes the psychiatric hospital as its own, and that a connection is made between an institution which is helping to rehabilitate people and a society which desires rehabilitation... Once the exclusionary nature of the traditional psychiatric institutions has been made clear towards the experimentation with new therapeutic dimensions, it is the external world which will determine the degree to which this new communication will be accepted.

(Franco Basaglia and Franca Ongaro, 'Introduction to Morire di classe', p. 6, cited in Foot, 2015, p. 357)

Giovanni Jervis, a colleague of Basaglia's, put it like this:

We wanted to see if it was possible to carry out psychiatric work in neighbourhoods, villages, hospitals, amongst the people, in the heart of the social fabric, and no longer at the asylum itself.

(Foot, 2015, p. 291)

Jervis went about things differently. He began to reform the psychiatric system in Reggio Emilia by establishing resources in society first, as a way to get people away from psychiatric hospitals. In other words, he began his work outside the institution and not from within it as in Gorizia. There, the hospital itself had been reformed first, by dismantling the unequal power relations between the healthcare workers and patients and setting up a therapeutic community. In other Italian locations too, such as Arezzo and Trieste, the process began not with the democratisation of the psychiatric system, but with the setting up of facilities outside the hospital. And this did allow people to get away from the institution.

Instead of focusing on 'the excluded', they focused on 'the excluder'. Consideration was now given to the places a person could turn to outside the psychiatric system, to hospitable places, and this is the work of the quartermaker. Quartermakers are concerned with the environment in which a patient arrives once he or she is discharged.

In 1978 the Italian parliament passed an act that led to the closure of its psychiatric institutions. That act is frequently referred to by the name of the psychiatrist who argued most vehemently for the hospital closures: Franco Basaglia.

September 2016. It is very sunny as we walk the grounds of the former hospital in Arezzo. We walk down a long path that gives a street-side view of the main building, the one with the clock high on the front wall. It must have towered over the patients and staff, as a reminder of time's passing. Or did it hasten patients to work in one of the buildings in the grounds? I suspect the latter.

The 'Manicomio Provinciale' in Arezzo has been closed since 1990. Of the former psychiatric hospital buildings, all but one, which still houses about ten patients, were taken by the university. Students now roam gardens that were once set aside for psychiatric patients. They sit on benches and talk. Agostino Pirella, a friend of Franco Basaglia's, oversaw the closure of the institution in the 1970s and brought mental healthcare into the community. We are visiting the present-day library, the 'Sala dei Grandi', where the first meetings, known as the 'General Assembly' were held between the patients and staff who introduced the democratisation of psychiatry in this very place. The decision to hold the meetings there must have been symbolic, given that the area was forbidden to patients prior to the reforms. On exiting the room we find Lucilla Gigli awaiting us. We get a two-hour, private guided tour of her institution records, a wonderful library of old psychiatric manuals and bound magazines and a room devoted to patient files. From one of the dossiers she shows us a letter, written by a woman to her psychiatrist. To her letter there is no reply. But the woman's medical records are there, along with observational notes of her behaviour. When the patient is unsettled, she is transferred to a pavilion for the 'troubled'. A stay of many years. The notes become fewer and further between as her stay progresses. Just one a year at times. A few words, merely to confirm that the patient is calm. Then, at the very end of the file, there is just a date, accompanied by a single word: 'idem'. Lucilla tells us about the work the patients did in the gardens and workshops. It was a hard life, isolated from family and friends. Many spent their lives here unnecessarily. We see paintings that were made in the hospital, as well as photographs, including one in which Pirella can be seen alongside Basaglia and Pasquale Spadi, a patient who frequently chaired meetings at the time of the reforms. 'Images of the revolution', says Lucilla with a smile, justifiably proud of this photograph. Pirella was the first to open the buildings to the neighbourhood's residents, by setting up a café on the grounds. It was the first time that patients and locals had a place to meet in the psychiatric institution. Each of the buildings retains its name from the days of the psychiatric institution, and there is a photograph on the front of each building showing some of the patients that lived or worked there. They really are prepared to draw a line here, and to move away from a past in which people with mental ill health were unfairly treated. Lucilla put together an exhibition about the dismantling of the institution. One of the exhibition's visitors recognised a photograph of his father. The father can be seen at a party organised by the patients and psychiatrists. The son never saw the father again after his admission. After seeing this photograph of his father the son contacted Lucilla and together they went through his father's records. An incredibly emotional experience for both of them. Apparently the closure of the hospital to visitors, family members included, left relatives resigned to the fact that they would never see each other again. The sorrow at parting persisted, it was traumatic, but it was never mentioned again. Until now. Lucilla tells us that for this reason alone the exhibitions and patient records are vital to the surviving relatives as they try to piece together their predecessors' histories. The pain is only exacerbated by the fact that these records reveal the lack of care with which the people who stayed here were treated.

We thank Lucilla warmly for the time she has set aside for us and especially for the kindness and compassion with which she talks about people with mental ill health. She is helping to ensure that people never forget what happened here.

In the grounds of the former institution stands a marble statue (sculpted by Matteo Maggio and Paolo Bacci) depicting a sitting girl on a plinth with two broken columns, the symbol of a life cut short. It is a monument in remembrance of the people who stayed there. It was unveiled on 28 March 2009 in honour of the victims of the psychiatric institution. The monument was designed not only as a reminder of the violence that was used in the institutions, but as a celebration of the patients' liberation from them. This monument, which is so clearly an apology for everything that went wrong in psychiatric institutions, is to my knowledge the only one of its kind in the world. It is an important monument, since the victims of psychiatry, the patients and their families, find it healing to see people in mental healthcare themselves recognise what went wrong, and what is going wrong. It is vital that the trauma experienced by these people as a result of their admissions be opened to discussion. An acknowledgement of what went wrong in psychiatry allows it to be spoken about, and for those who feel the need, such as healthcare professionals, family, patients and former patients, it allows them to grieve.

Article 107 (2002) sets in motion a gradual reduction in the number of psychiatric beds in Belgium. An important moment, because it is the first acknowledgement in centuries that an admission to hospital may not always be the best choice. For me, Article 107 is a call to search even harder for alternatives to psychiatric hospitals in their current form. Here, as opposed to Italy, the process of change looks like being a gradual one. It Italy there was a pivotal moment that marked a break with the past. There was no process of gradual change that led to the humanisation of psychiatry in Italy. In the Italy of the 1960s and 1970s it seems that the patients' situation was more harrowing than it was in Belgium at that time. Given the gradualness of the change here it feels like we lack the momentum to look back. But the process of deinstitutionalisation, and with it the fight against exclusion, could present us with the ideal opportunity to do this, and to issue an official apology on behalf of psychiatry in the form of a monument. This monument would be a way of acknowledging the suffering that patients and their families went through as the result of psychiatric admissions. It would ease the pain for many who have been traumatised by psychiatric treatment, but above all it would create space to talk about what went wrong, and what is still wrong. It is high time that caregivers in psychiatry were less defensive in the face of criticism over the use of force, then and now.

If psychiatry sets itself up as a positive science and confines itself, on the basis of a purely biomedical model, to locating the causes of mental ill health in the brain, it is in danger of ignoring the impact it actually has society. It would not be a good idea, as I see it, for psychiatry to regard itself as independent of society. Caregivers should therefore be concerned not only with mental ill health, but with the attitude a society adopts towards mental ill health. We are talking about the degree to which a society, in other words all of us, is hospitable to people with mental ill health. Now that long-term sufferers of mental ill health are once again recognised as citizens first and foremost, it is up to all citizens to allow those with mental ill health to take their place among them again, despite the tensions and frictions that this might cause. Keeping them isolated in institutions holds them in the position of second-class citizens. Quartermaking gives us ways to make society more accessible for people with mental ill health. It is not about changing the behaviour of people with mental ill health, but about how we ourselves change the environment so that people with mental ill health can take their place in it.

Quartermaking is a military term. A small detachment of the army walks ahead, to set up camp at a place where the majority of the force is headed. Safety and comfort are the main thing. The majority of the force arrives at that place without further effort. *Quartermakers* are people who walk ahead to create safe places in society for those who would like to connect to that society.

1994: *Kiosk* magazine is born on the rehabilitation ward, to improve communication between the psychiatric hospital and the community. The municipality is a part of one of the biggest municipalities in East Flanders. It has about 7,000 residents. The campus, just one part of a later Psychiatric Centre merger, is licensed for 195 beds. Interestingly, the campus is roughly in the middle of the municipality. Patients walk from the institution to the village square every day, where they mix with the local residents. On one of my visits to the local residents, someone tells me that he loves walking, but always drives to the coast for a walk. He never walks in the neighbourhood, because almost everyone on foot is a patient. He is afraid that if he goes walking the other local residents will identify him as a patient from the institute. This is why he never walks in his own neighbourhood. Conversations like these show us that there is quite a lot of prejudice against the patients, even in our own neighbourhood.

Not many Fridays have passed in the years between 1993 and 2008 when there hasn't been an editorial meeting of *Kiosk* magazine. A group of patients, former patients and staff members, all current members of the magazine's editorial staff, meet for an hour to discuss what the next bimonthly edition will look like. We brainstorm about subjects to cover and people to interview. It can be quiet, or cosy, or exuberant, or deadly serious, or highly structured and sometimes it can be chaotic. In short, whoever is

106

there at the time has a huge influence on what happens. Just spouting ideas. Some of the suggestions are taken up, others lie around waiting to be dealt with. Most the time our ideas, topics and suggestions far exceed the article space, leaving us no choice but to roll a few over to the next edition.

We suspect that creating our magazine runs into the same problems and challenges as any other magazine you might pick up at the newsagent's Who do we interview? What sections should *Kiosk* have? How do we reach our target audience? Is there anything coming up in the next couple of months that would be worth writing about? Who writes what? People have to be reminded to bring their articles in. Who will do the illustrations? Type the texts and do the layout? Meet the deadlines, in other words. Write a text for the website. Put up the posters. Sell the latest edition around the wards and outside the institution? Manage the subscription list. Send *Kiosk* out to the subscribers, and so on.

We use a big board at the editorial meeting to fill in the content for the different sections. People volunteer to write a piece, or to go out and get interviews. We have a 'Behind the Scenes' section, in which staff are interviewed about their area of expertise: doctor, nurse, cleaner, occupational therapist... In another section, 'What Fun We Had' we review some of the activities held in the hospital wards. We like to stay up to date. One of our *Kiosk* staff reads through the papers every day at the local newsagent's. The newsagent lets him copy interesting articles (often to do with psychiatry, mental healthcare or discrimination) and our reporter makes short summaries of the articles for the 'Newspaper Clippings' section.

Some patients write pieces of their own, which vary from concert reports and exhibition reviews to life stories. We have a series entitled 'The Grandmaster's Thoughts On...', which includes some offbeat pieces like the one arguing that Elvis is still alive and in hiding. We don't try to shelter the reader from our writers' internal logic, but allow them to experience it in all its rawness, beauty and poignancy. In every issue we try to balance news and developments in psychiatry with more light-hearted subjects on sports and hobbies. We also pay a lot of attention to disability and discrimination. The main areas of interest are solidarity and tolerance.

We like to give patients the chance to explore new social roles: *Kiosk* reporter might be one, or artist, to lift them out of the exclusive role of patient. Putting together a magazine involves so many different tasks and assignments: photographer, computer expert, illustrator, reporter... and this allows many to explore new social roles to the best of their ability. Everyone is invited to participate, based on interests, and, of course, strengths and abilities. We no longer differentiate between staff and patients. We are all *Kiosk* staff and that is how we present ourselves.

Jeroen is a reporter for *Kiosk*, and he writes about everything to do with psychiatry, especially the rights of the patient. He works three days a week and is known in the workplace for his scathing criticism of the rule bending. Much of this is in the sense of action through writing. He writes letter after letter to all kinds of authorities, like the Council of State, the Prime minister, and this causes quite a few tensions and concerns in the workplace. When he begins working for *Kiosk* (which he is very motivated and keen to do) he writes fewer and fewer personal letters of complaint about the workplace. Now, through *Kiosk*, he stands up for the downtrodden and, through our magazine, speaks out about all kinds of deplorable situations, like the mismanagement of the social security system. He finds that he is greatly appreciated by our readers, who encourage him to maintain this critical outlook. As a reporter, and a writer, he finds himself in a respected position which brings him not into direct conflict with his environment but brings him recognition. In other words his mission has not changed, but is much more socially acceptable. Ways of identifying, like being a member of the *Kiosk* staff, can have a stabilising effect. He feels good about working for us, precisely because of our critical outlook on society. He is a vital member of staff and highly respected by everyone. At his request we undertake a successful letter-writing campaign to get a young man with a mental disability out of prison. The boy's father comes to thank us at a *Kiosk* meeting. Our magazine also carries a report of this meeting. Our reporter is the centre of attention, and rightly so.

I am reminded too of the poet who is able, through *Kiosk*, get his poetry read through socially acceptable means, and, through *Kiosk*, to get closer to others by coming in off the sidelines. Prior to that, through his critical outlook, he was always an outsider. Through the magazine we offer a platform for like-minded social critics. It is our mission to come together for a little more solidarity and tolerance in the world, and quite a few patients can identify with that.

Kiosk is a magazine that focuses on social action for those who are powerless and excluded. Our staff feel good in this socially critical milieu. We manage to convert the fury, which was only expressible through psychosis before, into social action. At the same time we often see the psychotic element vanish from the content, precisely because the writer feels heard and has been given the opportunity to channel their anger through communication.

From the beginning to the present day we have enjoyed a collaboration with the culture centre in the municipality. The municipal council gives us free tickets to some performances. We do not see them as charity, but as 'press cards' for our reporters. If you go to a performance, you write a review. This gives us a pool of permanent culture reporters. The staff at the culture centre help us get interviews with the performers. A culture reporter can come into being because someone was given the opportunity to interview their idol.

I am at an evening meeting in the rehabilitation department. On behalf of *Kiosk* I am talking about what we do, and about forthcoming performances at Evergem culture centre.

> Johan is sitting beside me at the table. He looks at the poster for The Scene and says, repeatedly, for his own benefit, my benefit and the benefit of the others, that he won't be going. But then... he slides the poster closer and then away. It looks like he is talking to himself: 'I will, I won't...' He knows The Scene's music very well. In the past, before he was admitted, he went to gigs regularly. He hardly ever goes now, apart from a few weeks ago when he went to rock band Zornik in the Culture Centre on a free *Kiosk* ticket. Hilde, one of the people in charge there, told me that Johan left his seat during the performance a few times, to go to the toilet. He had to walk past the stage to get there and people were a little irritated. I ask Johan about this, and he tells me for the first time that a side effect of his medication is going to the toilet a lot, and that he finds it just as irritating to have to keep leaving his seat. With Johan's consent I tell Hilde, and she is immediately willing to exchange Johan's ticket for one nearer the toilet, so he won't disturb anyone by leaving his seat. To reassure Johan I go to The Scene with him. Johan, I, and another *Kiosk* reporter buy band T-shirts and go for a drink at the Culture Centre cafeteria. Going out together has created a bond between us. We become three fans of The Scene for the evening.

This is an illustration of quartermaking at work in a psychiatric ward. Let's run over it briefly again.

First and foremost, information comes into the ward. We look at existing organisations that may be of significance to people with mental ill health. At this time there is a lot going on in the area of healthcare and recovery, so that not even the healthcare professionals can distinguish the full range of provisions. We try to convey a large quantity of information, general information included, in a systematic way. We take our information from the papers and the television news, and examine it in more detail through *Kiosk*. We talk about the various types of accommodation and the organisations concerned with this. We also keep up to date on politics and culture.

Mostly, we identify the difficulties that long-stay psychiatric patients face when they try to reconnect with organisations outside the psychiatric system. We talk about how *Kiosk* can help. We talk about the events, exhibitions and interviews that we plan to do through *Kiosk*...

For a rather distrustful Johan the showing of the poster is an important element. He has plenty of time to read the information through and assure himself that a performance is coming up, and that it will be near the institution. The healthcare professional does not press him to participate or take action, so Johan is able discuss his interests voluntarily. This gives the healthcare professional an opportunity to listen to the patient's scope for identification.

At *Kiosk* we try incredibly hard to connect to the patients' desire. After years of detention these desires may have faded to the background.

The posters I bring for Johan remind him of earlier days, when he used to go to concerts. He knows a lot of The Scene's songs and is proud of the fact. Going to the concert reaffirms his identity as a fan. He shows this very clearly by wearing the tee-shirt.

When you try to encourage identification with a role other than patient, you have to remember to show willing by doing something in the patient's environment, for him/her and with his/her agreement. Empowerment on its own is not enough. Johan has been asked about his interests many times in intakes and talk therapies, only to be sent on training courses that seemed pointless or beyond his abilities, but more often than not he was left with the feeling that the courses wouldn't get him any closer to his goal, and so they weren't worth embarking on. These training courses merely reminded him of his role as a 'school pupil', which usually only comes with memories of failure.

In general, the strength of the patient's motivation to find a place other than 'patient in an institution' is a better indicator of whether or not he has the social skills needed to function in that place. It should not matter if the healthcare professional regards the patient's wishes as unrealistic. You just travel the road with him.

Observations on a ward have little or no value in predicting if a project will succeed outside the institution. A person who refuses to help with the washing up or to make the coffee on a psychiatric hospital ward can be the most conscientious of workers if asked to do the same in an organisation like Amnesty International. On the proviso that s/he is at least proud of his/her role at the institution and wishes to identify with its goals.

As a healthcare professional you are often looking for organisations that lie outside the healthcare and training circuit. It can be extremely difficult and complex at times, but it can also be very simple.

In Johan's example, our question was handled with spontaneity and enthusiasm by Hilde at the Culture Centre. The final obstacle to his not attending the performance had been removed. To this end it was necessary for me, with Johan's consent, to give her a minimal piece of information about Johan. Doing nothing and hiding behind a very strict interpretation of the rules of professional confidentiality can be harmful to the patient. Hilde and Johan have met, and they know where they stand with each other. As a healthcare professional you build a bridge that makes it possible for Johan to attend more performances in the future.

The 'Famous Fleming' section is always pretty special. Politicians, athletes, artists... all have been on a visit. Most that came to our ward thought they had been invited to give a talk, and that an audience would be there to listen to what they had to say. Afterwards, they were positive about the huge volley of questions that was fired at them. No, they hadn't realised that psychiatric patients were so engaged with what was going on around them. It is something else when patients get to meet their idols in person. It creates a dynamic on the ward that gives people a sense that something very special and exciting might happen. When people with mental ill health spend a long time in inpatient care, we often see them slip fully into the identity of patient. An interview with a famous Fleming of some sort can often help us discover traces of a patient's original interests. I remember clearly how a withdrawn and apathetic man became animated when questioning Fred Delcourt, a world-famous referee in the 1970s. It turned out that the patient had been a referee for years, but had preferred not to mention it. And how, when an interview with sports journalist, Ivan Sonck, was announced, a quiet old man started talking about the many marathons he had run. The interview questions were prepared at the editorial meeting. He came and did voluntary work for us, so we got coaching from a professional journalist for several years. We invite the local press to the interviews too, which helps get us coverage for our projects in the paper.

My best memories are of the famous Flemings who come out openly in our interviews about their own mental health problems. By doing so they lower the threshold and make it easier for our staff to talk about them.

We bear in mind that our magazine staff are not tied to the project, and we hope that it will give them a springboard to other projects which are entirely unrelated to psychiatry. We want to give our staff the best possible chance to put psychiatry behind them. For that reason it is the professional staff who ensure the continuity of *Kiosk*. In our meetings we often talk about prejudice and discrimination against people with mental ill health. 'Common sense is the collection of prejudices acquired by age eighteen'. This is a quotation commonly attributed to Einstein. With this at first sight very surprising statement he means that everything we assume to be 'ordinary', 'normal' and 'obvious' is actually based on the things we learnt by eighteen and stopped questioning after that. We are no longer aware that we are bristling with prejudice. Common sense is that which seems obvious to us, and it is in the obvious that prejudice lies.

Our many years on *Kiosk* have led us to the conclusion that psychiatric patients do indeed come up against discrimination. Some see psychiatric patients and former psychiatric patients as unstable and unreliable by definition.

The danger of being socially engaged with a group of long-stay mental health patients is that you, as a group, can get caught up in the idea that you are absolutely right about exclusion, and see the other as the cause. Every personal or group failure can be put down to the other, because the other has something against people from a psychiatric setting. This characterises the other as the villain, leaving you no other role but that of victim. If a group turns into a pressure group or a sort of union, you are in danger of adhering to an ideology, and when you adhere to an ideology you become a person who is no longer able to question himself. You have to be careful to avoid self-stigmatisation.

At one of our *Kiosk* meetings we mention a local bar. A person at the meeting tells us that he has been barred by the owner, and that the owner has something against psychiatric patients. Another patient tells us that he has not had a problem with the bar owner. By the end of the discussion it turns out that the man wasn't welcome because he had started a fight. By allowing the discussion to run its course and not capping it instantly with the word 'discrimination', we give the patient room to question his own behaviour, i.e., fighting. In the end, the discussion is about how to behave in a bar, and about how excessive drinking can lead to violence. It is far too easy to blame every fault or failure on the intolerance or prejudice of the other. Patients are not automatically unstable because they are patients, nor are they infallible because they are patients.

Discrimination against psychiatric patients exits, and we need to be aware of it. But it would be wrong to say that discrimination is always present. That in itself would be a judgement. It only leads to self-stigma. We want to hold judgements like these up to scrutiny.

We want to be more than just socially critical. By organising parties, exhibitions, discussion evenings...we want to give a picture of life in a psychiatric hospital, and, above all, we want to show that there is no such thing as the typical psychiatric patient.

4.2 A Dramatic Turn

In the mid-1990s, amid plans to build a container park in the area, the local residents launched a protest campaign. Their main concern was the noise and traffic it would bring. We took part in the protest through *Kiosk* and were invited to a talk by the mayor. The municipal authorities listened to our complaints. Our engagement on the community's behalf increased our popularity with the local residents in an instant.

Kiosk also focused attention on the 'How Different Is Different' project run by the Flemish Association for Mental Health. Three times a year we welcomed several final and pre-final year students from a variety of schools to the ward for a few days, where they participated in the activities with the patients. On those occasions we had *Kiosk* meetings with the pupils and talked about prejudice and stigma and how to get around these. Three days are hardly enough to give a true picture of a psychiatric ward, but it is a start. Joka, the youth camp organisers, brought youngsters for their summer camp. They stayed on the ward for a week and organised all kinds of activities to create a holiday atmosphere. We took part in mini-football tournaments and other sports activities in the community. On two occasions a *Kiosk* football team (mostly patients from the other wards) played in mini-football tournaments in Evergem.

Many of patients who shop here, go to the football... would love to stay on and live in municipality. But sky-high rental prices make it virtually impossible, and social housing is in very short supply. Employment is another reason why few patients stay in the municipality. Through *Kiosk*, and an excellent partnership with the municipal council, we try to address these issues.

A few weeks before the election we always hold a debate, and we invite politicians from the different parties. We try to persuade patients to vote, essentially by asking questions of particular interest to them. We also ask the hospital psychiatrists not to be too quick to issue sick notes. In the first place patients are citizens, and in this country every citizen has a duty to vote. We also organise exhibitions to reach out to the local residents. One of these exhibitions is in collaboration with local artists and galleries. When an exhibition-related event takes place in the Culture Centre, professional writers and poets and people with mental health issues come and read passages from their own work. There is also a fashion show, at which patients take to the catwalk. A turn in the spotlight, literally, does the power of good.

In 2002, through the Festive Flanders initiative, the Flemish community sponsors neighbourhood parties for the first time, and we host a garden party at the psychiatric centre for our neighbourhood. We share the task of organising it with the local residents. We invite local organisations to come and present themselves by setting up stands on the grounds. Local sports clubs demonstrate table tennis, chess, rope skipping... There is a jumble sale. A marching band goes around the festival and there is a bouncy castle, pony rides and cooking classes for the kids... Party games are organised by Red Cross volunteers. Patients, local residents and members of staff give joint performances, handle the preparations, man the bar, wait on tables, enjoy the party, do the washing up and clear up the mess together afterwards. The day ends with a giant barbecue. These annual family festivals on a Sunday afternoon are always very successful.

We invite the press to these activities to spread word of what we do on a grander scale, and to give a broader, more realistic picture.

Just when we made all the preparations for our third annual neighbourhood party, a drama unfolds...

2004. When distant events take place, but have a very immediate effect on your life, you tend to remember exactly what you were doing at the time, even years afterwards. On the evening of Friday the 25th of June a colleague calls me at home with the news that a former patient has shot two local residents dead. The victims are a woman and her son. At the time of the call I am making a few preliminary sketches for a painting. I can still see the table and sheet of paper in front of me. Yellow flowers, tiny yellow flowers and the rest blank. Only when I watch the news that evening does the full force of the story begin to dawn on me. I see a short report on the murders. I see images of the chip shop I know and love so well, where something horrific, the unthinkable, has happened. Something irreversible has taken place. A (former) psychiatric patient has shot and killed two chip shop owners opposite the hospital. A passing cyclist was hit in the hand. The next day, a Saturday, I drive to the municipality very early in the morning. I remember contacting a police officer I had spoken to the week before in relation to his role in the upcoming neighbourhood party. He too is stunned. I meet with patients and local residents, and continue to do so in the days that follow. Talking, listening, consulting, welcoming people in... I reach out to anyone and everyone who is prepared to talk about the event. Meetings with the management. Consultations over the best way to deal with this, and a realisation that nothing more can be done than reach out and connect. In the hypervigilant state that comes in the weeks after the event there are several more reports of new dangers, which turn out, fortunately, to be false alarms.

There is only a very small distance between the hospital, the chip shop, the neighbourhood houses and the places where the former patient used to sleep. Needless to say, the incident causes a serious commotion. The police are called into question for allowing a rough sleeper to roam the neighbourhood for so long without intervening. And the psychiatric institution is called into question, since it was a former psychiatric patient who committed the murders.

In a few of the local shops patients experience stigmatisation first hand. One patient, standing in the queue, is simply bypassed by others, and the shopkeeper turns a blind eye to the queue jumpers. No one speaks out in the patient's defence. In the meantime, the hospital staff and patients lay flowers by the chip shop. The criticism continues. A group of people forms and takes a stand against the management. Then they go against the hospital and everyone in it. Reference is made to previous problems with patients in the neighbourhood, which some local residents claim the hospital has never addressed. A tense game of 'us and them' emerges. The local residents versus the people admitted for care.

After the funeral we hold a joint emergency meeting with the police in a room in a local café. Emotions run high, and many in the neighbourhood are saying that they no longer feel safe: "They are aggressive, they deal drugs, they walk the streets drunk, or stoned ..." Some believe that it would be in the best interests of the patients to keep them within the grounds of the institution. It is dangerous for them on the street. They are not always aware of the danger posed by the traffic in this area. People use the same argument to separate patients from local residents by talking about how beautiful the hospital garden is. They see the garden as the place for patients and the street as the place for the local residents. The counter argument, that reduced mobility is no reason to keep a physically disabled person away from the road, does not go down well.

What will stay with me forever is a remark by a man who calmly and quietly asserts that he isn't afraid of patients who are recognisable by their odd behaviour, because he can always cross the street when he sees them, but that he is particularly uneasy about the idea of people walking around who are not recognisable as patients. He suggests that they be given a sign or a mark by which local residents will be able to recognise them. Obviously, the feeling of being unsafe leads to more stigmatisation. This brings the original meaning, the basic meaning of the word to the surface: to mark the body with a sign by which the lesser person, the different person, the person to be avoided can be recognised.

> stigma was defined as bodily signs designed to expose something unusual and bad about the moral status of the signifier.
>
> (Goffman, 1990, p. 11)

At the first meeting with local residents it was difficult for the health-care professionals to maintain that people with mental ill health are not generally dangerous: this extreme act of violence had taken place before our very eyes. Only a handful of people among the two-hundred-strong crowd made any attempt to keep things calm. At a point when the hospital itself comes under fire, a few local residents say that anyone could find themselves needing to be admitted, and that you can never tell in advance. In the face of the clamour a doctor says: "You should not be so hasty in your desire to close the hospital; in this hectic society every one of us is a potential patient. There is a very good chance of us having to call on a service, like psychiatry, at some point." It was clear that the only purpose of an emotionally charged meeting like this – which was also attended by the family of the deceased – could be to allow people to vent their feelings, to listen to people in shock. We were very clearly on the defensive, and we took a very understanding approach. It was my first live experience of a situation in which people, expressing the most horrendous prejudices through emotion, have to be heard before any real discussion can take place.

The young man who rode past at the time of the murders in June 2014, and was hit in the hand, gets in touch with me. He would love to come to the ward and tell the patients that he is not in agreement with local residents who now regard all patients as dangerous. He does not wish to come across as being in any way prejudiced towards psychiatric patients, even after this terrible experience with a mentally ill person, and wants to come and say this. He wants to tell us that he does not view all people with mental ill health as violent. We arrange a meeting with the patients, at which he can tell his story. He lets it be known that he does not subscribe to the 'us and them' idea, 'us' being the local residents and 'them' being the patients. This becomes something of a motto, stretching across everything we later accomplish in the community. 'Us' stands for every local resident, and that includes the patients and staff at the psychiatric institute. We work as a team to keep the neighbourhood safe and hospitable. The neighbourhood, and life in the neighbourhood, is dear to us.

After the event we began by trying to accommodate people's emotions, by listening to them first and only then responding. Our hospital directors went for a far-reaching, structural partnership with the local community based on a care hotline and consultation platform. They are both in existence to this day.

> (free translation) The care line should be seen as an example of an infrastructure that helps citizens live with discord. It acknowledges the difference of the patient as well as the position of fellow citizens.
>
> (Kal, 2001, p. 168)

Our care hotline follows a rigorous, step-by-step plan and has given good results. People can get through on the reception telephone number or by email. Every incoming message is recorded in writing and, of course, taken seriously. A member of the hospital staff attends the scene immediately, listens to the problem and resolves it there and then if possible. Sometimes a complainant will discover that the person they have reported is not an inpatient. In such cases we refer them to other services for further assistance. Complainants are also notified any further action taken at a later date. Staff at the psychiatric centre perform a weekly evaluation of incoming and processed complaints. An analysis is made of the complaints. And an assessment is made of how the complaints were handled.

The aim is to lower the communication barriers between the psychiatric system and the local community. By taking every complaint seriously you leave the door ajar. Doortje Kal puts it like this: (free translation) 'You can only expect your neighbourhood residents to be there for your patients if you and your staff are there for your neighbourhood residents' (Kal, 2001, p. 167).

Along with the hotline, a quarterly meeting of hospital staff and local residents was set up. This consultation platform ultimately became a core group of about 15 volunteers, represented by people living in the vicinity of the hospital, associations in the neighbourhood and hospital staff, as well as local politicians and the local police. For the local residents it is all about avoiding patient nuisance: resolving problems as and when they arise, or preventing them in the first place, and passing on information about how the process works. For the psychiatric centre's patients and staff it is all about de-stigmatising patients, to pave the way for reintegration into society. The meetings are also used to encourage people from the neighbourhood to participate in our neighbourhood projects.

The complaints range from reports of a person seen wandering the streets aimlessly to, on one occasion, a case of serious vandalism. The local storekeeper occasionally complains about alcohol misuse outside the store or theft. The number of complaints is stable, at about two a month. There is an arrangement with the police to pass the complainants' details on for the more serious matters. We don't run the hotline to assist the police, but through a desire to be there for our local residents if they are prepared to be there for our patients, through good and bad. We want to be there for them if they don't know how to respond to a patient's behaviour. Through this work we can sometimes make seemingly odd behaviours a little easier for others to understand and combat prejudice and stigma.

Frequent contact with local residents gives us an understanding of how local residents think and allows us to relay more targeted information about living and working in the institution, to help dispel any misunderstandings.

A group of patients with an escort can convey the mistaken idea that the patients are dangerous. Local residents assume that the escort is there for the residents' safety. If the escort is a female nurse on her own, this way of thinking can make it look like we are going light on security. It is important for us to let local residents know that escorts are not always there for safety, but that we just see it as a part of our job to get out and about with our patients.

> Early one morning a report comes in of a woman walking the streets in pyjamas. A local resident calls in to say that someone has escaped the ward. On looking into the matter we were able to inform the local resident that the lady in question likes to wear pyjamas because she is comfortable in them, and that she is staying on an open ward. The local resident reported the matter having incorrectly assumed that all the wards were secure, and that a person wandering around in pyjamas so early in the morning must have escaped. Investigating reports like these can help us rectify a few misconceptions. We were able to tell him that most wards are open, and that people with mental health issues are free to walk in and out unchecked.

The reports can be tackled in this way to reduce stigmatisation among the local residents. The idea that many of the patients are dangerous, that they are locked up and that they might escape, is one that we do occasionally come across.

We remind the patients that we are in partnership with the neighbourhood, and that living in a neighbourhood in which everyone looks after each other is one of our concerns, and should also be one of theirs. Local residents also have a part to play in making life more liveable in the neighbourhood: when shopkeepers remove the alcoholic drinks from their automatic dispensers, for example. This, along with more vigilance on the wards, helped lower the number of alcohol-related complaints in the neighbourhood. At consultation platform meetings the local police officer tells us that, where statistics are concerned, social problems in this neighbourhood are no higher than in any other. This shows the complaints in a wider perspective and puts them into context. Fact-checking the information has a destigmatising effect. In other words, the area around the psychiatric centre is an entirely normal neighbourhood, with plenty of opportunity for pleasant encounters and its fair share of conflicts and problems.

Within this structure, our *Kiosk* magazine is an important incubator for ideas and projects to promote integration. Feedback comes through to us on this from the consultation platform. By discussing our projects on the consultation platform we raise awareness among local residents of opportunities to take part in actions to promote the integration of our target group.

Some local residents bake cakes when we organise an activity. Others man the reception desks at the exhibitions we hold. When the local shopkeeper decides to retire, we invite him to come and say his goodbyes at the hospital. A local bee keeper always gives me a warm welcome, and I take patients with me when I visit. There are rabbits, frogs and birds of all kinds to be seen...We are always given a tour of the garden, to see the animals. The patients bring scraps of bread for this local resident, to feed the animals.

Organisations from the neighbourhood can ask us for an information pack about the institution. In that case we describe the activities of the various wards and put them in touch with members of the *Kiosk* staff. This gives patients the opportunity to tell the visitors about themselves.

Setting up connections calls for a little creativity, but it generates a great deal of warmth and affinity between people, whatever their backgrounds.

The consultation platform has been going for some 15 years, and we still come across locals who are unaware that the meetings take place. Some local residents come for the first time after experiencing an issue with a patient. They are welcomed by others who have been attending the group meetings for a while, and the old hands tell the newcomers how it all works. They soon convert the indignation to cooperation. When we get angry newcomers I arrange to visit them at home. On one of these visits a resident tells me about a patient who shadow boxes his way down the street, and he asks me if the man is violent. Looking at the street from the resident's window I can imagine that I too would be inclined to stay in when this shadow-boxer comes by. Working at the hospital as I do, I know the patient, and I know that he wouldn't hurt a fly. But the local resident doesn't know him, and doesn't have enough contact for a proper assessment of the threat. I think it is important to let the resident know that there is no need to be afraid of this shadow-boxer. Meeting is the important thing, but to be able to, or to have the courage to, can sometimes require intermediaries or mediators. It is important for the people living around the institution to have people at the institution who they trust. Members of staff, who act as mediators. Hardly a new idea.

Residents who have been here a long time tell me about the old relationship between the hospital and the local community. The hospital garden was a favourite afternoon walk for many residents. They would come to see the aviaries of exotic birds. There would be cows grazing on the grass in front of the entrance. The garden was like a public park, where they would also come across patients. Back then there was a lot of greenery, and there were paths to walk on, which made it feel safe. Children would hide in the park to skip school. There would be the odd commotion if the locals saw someone wandering around naked. And there were the terrible moments when a body would be found in one of the canals around the grounds. After several suicides the walls were taken down. People from the municipality used to attend mass in the hospital chapel. The garden was one of the local wedding photographer's favourite backgrounds. On what was supposed to be the most beautiful day of their lives, generations of residents were immortalised in photo albums, in the garden, with the psychiatric hospital behind them. Long before today's community work became a profession, the friars performed the task without ever really being aware of it. They were well known in the village. They actually lived in the institution and were always available. Through the professionalisation, the downsizing of the gardens (for a larger staff car park) the more rapid changes in patient population (more addiction issues) many of the meeting places and opportunities for encounters between the local community and the institution disappeared. And with them disappeared the friars, or the points of contact. Their social task, which they had not originally conceived as a task, but as a natural development, is now in need of professionalisation and has become the task of the quartermaker. Whereas the garden was once a lovely spot to come for a walk on a Sunday, we find ourselves trying to attract local residents to the institution by other means. There is the fitness trail in the garden, and there are the sports halls, which organisations from the area sometimes use. We need other strengths to make the institution more attractive to the local community.

We have united patients and local residents in a few litter campaigns. We have organised a thematic information evening, involving films and exhibitions. Since we considered ourselves to be on the right track, and justifiably so, we entered the national 'Lilly Reintegration Award' competition for projects in support of social reintegration for psychiatric patients. Our community outreach programme (Hotline, Consultation Platform and *Kiosk*) was selected as the best Belgian project in 2006 and we scooped the Lilly Reintegration Award. When we took to the stage with local residents and patients to accept the prize in front of a packed cinema hall on Mental Healthcare Day, it was an extraordinarily beautiful moment. The jury report talked about the courage and perseverance we had shown as a community and an institution by establishing a partnership of this kind in the wake of such a terrible event. We were proud to have achieved this together. And with the prize money we could organise new community initiatives.

4.3 Citizen Friendships

In Hans Reinders' footsteps, Doortje Kal talks about citizen friendship: (free translation) 'Citizen friendship exists wherever citizens are fellow citizens to each other; they share in each other's lives so that each can prosper' (Kal, 2001, p. 26).

Citizen friendships arise in different ways through our projects.

A local organises two cycling trips every year. He works out a route and arranges meetings with interesting people on the way. In fact we always mix business with pleasure and make every encounter something of a celebration in its own right.

We reimagine our annual neighbourhood party by organising a jumble sale and a bike and wagon tour. Through 'Love Your Neighbourhood' we invite local residents in for coffee, and to usher in the new year the volunteers invite us to a party, for the sixth year now, at which we, the staff and the patients celebrate the new year with other local residents. It is remarkable, when watching people with mental ill health in contact with others, how you begin to notice their deeply buried qualities and strengths. In Mark's case, it is the disarming manner in which he relates to people he doesn't know. He appears, through his rather naive and friendly way of approaching people, to bring happiness and good cheer. In his company, people seem less formal and awkward with each other. I have heard a local resident say something similar. He was talking about a man with mental ill health who, through his manner and presence in the shop, managed to get customers interacting in a very open and friendly way. There was something about the man's spontaneity that got people responding, not just to him, but to each other, in a more spontaneous way.

The vast majority of the community activities we are involved in originate from organisations that rely on the municipal authority: the culture centre, public centre for social welfare...

Political views, such as that excessive government interference undermines citizens' ability to care for one another, or alternatively, the opinion that everything should be in the hands of the state so that people can truly care for each other, do not add up. It is my feeling that both, i.e. local political and community initiatives, are best applied hand in hand. For that reason it is very important for the quartermaker to be in touch with the local politicians. In this way there is a collaboration necessary to these politicians about necessary changes in the neighbourhood.

Kiosk has developed a platform for social action, a place from which we organise workshops or open days for the community and do even more specific work in the area of quartermaking. We have put ourselves forward to the municipal authority as an organisation that aims to care for the community. In exchange for this work, which the municipality also views as community social work, the municipality has given us free use of premises on Cardijnwijk, a few hundred metres away from the psychiatric hospital. We use it for meetings with local residents. Local politicians can play a facilitating role in the community for quartermakers from the psychiatric hospital.

Our location within the community itself makes us more accessible. This location is a 'shared space', which increases our chance of meeting other neighbourhood residents and organisations. The fact that we no longer meet in the hospital makes it easier for former patients to stay connected without feeling like patients, and we are more accessible for local residents who would like to join us. A few are still afraid to come into the actual hospital.

One of the finest *Kiosk* projects on the integration of (former) psychiatric patients in the community has been the poetry trail. We asked (former) patients from a number of institutions, patient organisations, half-way houses and day centres to write poems about home and about mental ill health.

In the winter prior to the project we, the staff, a few local residents and some (former) patients went door-to-door in the community, asking locals if they would post a poem by a former patient in their window for two months. We got an enthusiastic response. More than a hundred households participated and many of the poems stayed up after the two months had passed. The poems were posted in the windows of people's homes along a route from the hospital to the site of our weekly Cardijnwijk gathering. These are two places that prize the idea of hospitality. By this means the route from the hospital to the community centre became a hospitable place in itself. Walking down the street and looking at the windows, where we see our poems, we get the sense that we are welcome here in this community. Art is a way of connecting, of connecting with the residents of this area, an area to which we belong. It improves social cohesion. We work on the assumption that a hospitable area is one where being different is also welcomed.

Three of the poems were enlarged and displayed permanently as part of the street scene on the hospital railings. At the event itself patients read their poems aloud and collections of poetry were sold. Through its enthusiasm for this work the municipality has expressed solidarity with the idea that (former) patients are citizens too, and that they are entitled to a home in the community. We are bringing people out of the psychiatric system and into the public space. We are demonstrating that these people may be different, but above all, people, with the same ideas and wishes as others outside the institution.

The chip shop stands on a railway-owned site (Nationale Maatschappij der Belgische Spoorwegen) and, 12 years on from the murders, it is in a state of disrepair. The broken windows, ripped posters and dilapidation do a disservice to the memory of the people who were killed there. Of its own accord the municipal authority finally decides to clear the site. A participation project is set up in tandem with our Consultation Platform. Local residents are invited to contribute ideas for the site. The family of the victims is also asked to participate. A demolition date for the chip shop is agreed.

14 October 2015. A grey and chilly morning. A few locals stand on the footpath beside the chip shop. I, and a few colleagues and patients, walk over and stand beside them. The demolition crew is fencing off the site. By signalling that the site is no longer safe to enter, the fences only add to the sense of desolation. But they are also a sign that something is about to happen. The demolition crew are aware of our reasons for saying farewell to the site again. Local residents remember Jurgen and Nadine once more. They were much loved in the community. For the last time we look at what was once the chip shop. A huge skip has been brought in for the rubble. A couple of the victims' relatives, whom we now know, come across to greet us. They stand very close to the fencing. People take photos or videos of the demolition. We are aware of the significance of the moment. It is the next step in the healing process. With every bite, the grab crane rips the chip shop apart. The debris rises high in the air before dropping into the skip. Someone cries, quietly. After everything has gone, a sense of relief. The gradual decline of this place had been painful to watch. It has created new room and space, literally and figuratively: room and space for something new. We are free once more to think ahead about this space, to give it a new purpose without forgetting the past. On the evening prior to the demolition there is a meeting of the consultation platform, attended by some 40 local residents, the hospital staff and the mayor and aldermen. We discuss the new designation for this place. The local residents produce drawings and designs. Several meetings follow, attended by the NMBS and a delegation of provincial officials. The railway company intends to build a passenger car park on the site, and the provincial authorities want to plan the start of a cycle path. With the mayor's help we manage to set a portion of the land aside for our community project. A few months later, in June 2016, it is made official. The local residents, hospital staff and patients will get a say in the future use of the land. It becomes a community space, a place of rest and a place of commemoration, where the central idea is that of the meeting place. Where 'us' and 'them' are put aside and replaced with 'we', meaning the people of this community. It makes no difference whether you live, work or stay at the hospital here. This very place, with its terrible history, will be a place of hope and cooperation. The building blocks for the project are openness, meeting, appealing

to young and old, greenery, commemoration, maintenance-friendliness and participation by local residents and people from the psychiatric hospital.

We meet in the council chamber in October 2016: the municipal authority, local residents, patients and members of the hospital staff. It is an important and symbolic meeting, a beginning. The people from the municipal authority allow our group a sum of money with which to complete the site. The municipal authority creates opportunities for inclusive cooperation. The land will belong to us, to the community, a hospitable community, a community of solidarity. We plan a covered meeting space with a book-exchange cabinet, a bug hotel, a petanque court and an exhibition wall. There will also be a remembrance space. As you can imagine, there is a relationship between being preventive and offensive in your promotion of social integration, and being reactive and defensive. The more preventive you are, the better your chances of being offensive. By being offensive, I mean taking hold of the reins and deciding where your priorities lie. You decide your own agenda.

Being preventive places a vast range of options at your disposal for quartermaking. At a particular point, the murders in the community forced us to be reactive and defensive, which meant that for many years the priority was safety, and rightly so. The community set very high demands when it came to safety, quite understandably, and the institution had to find a response. This slowed our work on stigmatisation and social integration. But we have always seen the two as linked. The complaints that came in through the consultation platform had to be dealt with, in collaboration with the local police, but we continued to give local residents the opportunity, through the actions we organised, to lend a hand when it came to integrating patients in the community. We view the combination of safety and cooperation as a strength.

This defensive attitude is extremely difficult, even impossible to drop. Some 12 years after the murders, when the community and I asked for coverage of our collaboration on the community square, the regional broadcaster aired a clip of the news bulletin at the time of the murders. At the end of the interview, the reporter seemed to apologise for rebroadcasting these images. He said that while, ultimately, it is a very fine example of collaboration, we also need to focus attention on the terrible event that took place. The wonderful collaboration story is linked to the horror of what happened on that spot. For that reason, commemoration will always be an essential element. Collaboration with the families of the people who died is also extremely important. These elements produced a situation in which the psychiatric hospital developed a neighbourhood project which is one of a kind in Belgium and The Netherlands.

Being more preventive (in mental healthcare and in society) can make projects on destigmatisation more effective. This preventive approach is realised through closer and better cooperative ties with organisations in and outside the mental healthcare setting.

Through contact with the various local authorities, we discovered more ways to collaborate with local residents. These activities have now been incorporated in the ward programme, which we offer to people on admission.

On the rehab ward, we try to base as many activities as we can on meetings. We have stopped calling these activities therapies, because we want to normalise relations between healthcare professionals, patients and local residents. Cooking, creative activities, music... We are forever looking at how to organise things in a way that gets others involved. The diversity of our contact with citizens allows us to cater to the capacities and interests of anyone who would like to volunteer for us. At present, the folk at the Red Cross also prefer group activities to buddy contacts.

Our fellow staff on the ward see themselves as community workers as well as hospital employees. Having one foot in the ward and one in the community allows us to build bridges between the ward and the community. It ensures that people who stay on the ward can also be in contact with people from the local environment. We aim to do everything we can to lift people out of their social isolation by opening the ward to outsiders.

4.4 Basic Elements of Quartermaking

When I mention quartermaking most people tell me that, although they understand what I mean, they cannot exactly explain what it is. Going out on walks makes people stronger and more vigorous. That's a very good thing. Patients get a new lease on life by getting away from the ward. But quartermaking is another thing altogether.

You get to work on a patient's dreams and expectations. As a healthcare professional you try to help them realise these dreams. You try to find supporters to help you along the way. It is a creative journey, full of trial and error, which some colleagues describe as 'unrealistic'. And they sometimes add that the job of the healthcare professional is to bring a sense of reality to the patient and, through therapy, to grieve for unfulfilled expectations. Often there is no need to convey a sense of reality to patients. They are no strangers to life's harsh realities. The good thing is that they at least have dreams. Networking, and quartermaking in general, is a very realistic way to actually achieve some of the goals. It works, if you take the trouble to work at it yourself. And, above all, it takes you from healthcare provider to hope provider, an extremely powerful element in your contact with the people you treat.

Quartermaking is not an ideology. It is a work method that is used to achieve integration on the basis of a patient's wishes at a particular time and place. Something else may have to be done at a later stage. It is a means of integration. Quartermaking is a necessary intermediate step that should, ideally, render itself superfluous. Doortje Kal's work is not always an easy read, but the quartermaker who sticks with it will be all the richer for the experience. The claim of her thesis is that:

> (free translation) The attempt to socially integrate people with a psychiatric background confronts the receiving society with discord. To support integration that does not culminate in unilateral assimilation it is necessary to create space for the strange other, as a part of which it should be accepted that this other will remain strange to some extent and therefore 'inconvenient'. This action of 'creating space for' is explained by the concept of quartermaking. In allowing access for and to the strange other, quartermaking is suitable as an intermediate step: the normal run of things must be suspended and turned to an object of reflection, due to that which is not commonplace in society.
>
> (Kal, 2001, pp. 28–29)

I often find statements that emphasise the universality of being human, the fact that we are all recovering, that we are all beings who search for meaning. While it is all well and good to generalise mental health issues as a part of being human, this also implies that people with such issues do not exist as a group. It places the emphasis on our similarity, the fact that in the end we all have the same ideas and feelings. We are almost literally asked to ignore the differences. This can be exceptionally difficult at times, and it can be uncomfortable if a person's suffering is so great that they sense a huge distance between themselves and others who suffer less. If we say things like 'we are all the same' and 'everyone is flawed' there is a good chance of the person feeling we are not taking their suffering seriously. They might feel that they are being asked to stop moaning, because we all have a tough time of it sometimes. Although one person's suffering cannot really be compared to another's, it seems to me that the suffering of the person who hear voices or has delusions, is of a different order of magnitude to that of the person who does not really want to get out of bed in the morning.

One reason for distinguishing our target group as a separate group, is that people with mental ill health are discriminated against. If you have been in an institution for a long time it is harder to find a home to rent, harder to find a job. If we stop calling the group a group, we will not be able to talk about discrimination against them, which would mean not being able to do anything about that discrimination. Acknowledging the grey areas means that as well as recognising the huge importance that we attach to our shared humanity, our universal vulnerability, whilst daring to bring differences into relief.

Doortje Kal does not accept that citizens do not feel any connection with people with mental ill health or that people with mental ill health belong in places where they can live together in seclusion ... (free translation) 'The acceptance of discord is extremely important, and this is the acceptance that a return from the psychiatric system creates tensions' (reference to the anti-psychiatry movement, Ibid., pp. 36–37).

Acceptance of difference sets up a tension that we should not try to resolve. A space should be set aside for difference.

Rudi Visker talks about this in his book, *Vreemd gaan en vreemd blijven*

> (free translation) A racist reduces the other to the colour of his skin. The anti-racist counter to this is that skin colour is not an issue. He is wrong (...) because for a person with skin colour the issue of skin colour is precisely that there is something about us and we don't know what it means, but that it plays a role nonetheless, just as our gender, the meaning of which we do not know, plays a role and possibly more than the things to which we attach importance and the meaning of which we do know.
>
> Acknowledging the other regardless of his skin colour, saying that the colour does not matter, is depriving him of the question to which he himself has no answer, but which he does not wish to lose because he derives not only his suffering but his worth from that which is not public for him. What I say about skin colour here also applies to other forms of difference that make the person who they are. These differences escape the grasp of the person they differentiate. Like gender, skin colour is a form of transcendence that does not speak. A person's worth is to do with something that is silent, a dumb transcendence.
>
> (Visker, 2005, p. 318)

The nice thing about this piece is that it stresses the fact that as a person we are strange to ourselves. That we are not whole, but alien to ourselves. Our body, for example, is alien to us, alien to our thoughts. We do not know what happens inside our body. We feel pain and joy, but have no way of telling what goes on in our body. In this sense our body is strange to us. We have characteristics that we cannot control. We can consider them, have ideas about them, but our own reactions can often take us by surprise.

Space for the *strange Other*. With these words Doortje Kal (2001) refers to the work of Luce Irigaray, who sought to develop a philosophical theory of the strange Other, primarily the woman in her case (Irigaray, 1992). She did not wish to identify a universal subject. For her, the *strange Other* is the woman and this is what she calls her. The emphasis is on the difference. It is about not being afraid to categorise people as different, as this allows us to talk about the space to be created for these people. When we look for a universal subject by erasing the differences, the term equal takes on the sense of identical, instead of the much more important one of equivalent in value.

Doortje Kal looks for an exposition in which the other can appear as 'other'. (free translation) 'In brief, the categorisation is used by quartermakers to identify people with psychiatric problems through their difference, without them having to pay for it through confinement or exclusion' (Kal, 2001, p. 27). The ideal of being identical would compel people with mental ill health to reflect and match the picture of an assumed normality. Becoming identical in this way could only be oppressive. Terms such as 'difference' and 'equivalence in value' can complement each other, as can 'normality' and 'equality'. Creating an absolute normality forces people to assimilate before they can belong to the group. They must become what is expected of them, a person who thinks, feels and behaves like people who are regarded as 'normal'.

So while there are different groups of people, this does not mean that they should be kept apart because some live in an institution and others do not. We are not at one with ourselves. Recognising the strangeness in ourselves should help us appreciate the strangeness of the other.

In this sense, the word 'compassion' is interesting. The Old Dutch word 'doghen' means 'suffering' and occurs in the word 'gedo-gen' (meaning 'to tolerate'). And this is how we arrive at the meaning of permitting or tolerating. Strange behaviour can be irritating to anyone who watches it. It comes across as abnormal, and therefore disturbing. There is something incomprehensible about it, and it can be frightening for that reason. We cannot put it into context. It disturbs the normal order of things.

Having compassion means seeing people not in terms of good or bad. Acknowledging and accepting our own excessive impulses, which we ourselves find surprising and alienating, allows us to comprehend the strange impulses of others. Compassion reveals the other as human, despite his strange or negative characteristics, as a result of which a meeting can always take place. Compassion differs from pity in that it is not based on appreciation for the suffering, but appreciation for a mix of wrongdoing and being wronged, for the immense complexity that often binds the two.

By noticing and acknowledging the difference, the other in ourselves, we can open ourselves to the difference in the other. This acknowledgement, this setting aside of a space and meeting each other within it, without trying to iron out differences, is what quartermaking is all about.

But in this sense we, as quartermakers, can also have compassion for local residents who feel troubled by, and have a tendency to exclude, people with mental ill health. It is compassion that allows us to be present not only with patients, but also with these local residents, in the hope that they will change their feelings, thoughts and behaviour towards this *strange Other*. Compassion allows us to appreciate both sides in a quarrel or confrontation, and to try to mediate from that position.

We can often tolerate something in someone else if we understand it through this kind of acknowledgement. Finding explanations for behaviours that seem strange at first can be reassuring, but acknowledging them can give way to compassion. There is always more than one explanation.

You talk about a person's very idiosyncratic logic, with a view to bringing that logic, which was very obscure at first, out into the open. Doortje Kal calls this a suspension of the conventional. Reinterpreting normality through the patient's logic (Ibid., pp. 62, 63, 116).

> Francis is on a work training scheme. It's going really well. The training supervisors in the workplace are very pleased. The training supervisors at college are pleased. But then he suddenly stops coming to work. He is absent several times and ignores the reminders. No one can get in touch with him, not even the FACT Team. Reference is made to his illness, his diagnosis provides an explanation for his absence. The practical implications of this illness are that he cannot sustain a course of action, and that he fails repeatedly. It is a fatalistic, circular argument. Fatalistic, because the environment gives up on him. The supervisors appear to be lacking in compassion and wish to remove him from the training scheme. It has a long waiting list, and there are plenty of people on the list who actually 'are' motivated to get a job. When I was counselling him at home he spoke about his relationship with his family. His mental health issues are due to his being given at a very tender age the responsibility for looking after and supporting his brothers and sisters. His parents made a bad job of it. Even now, he does not want his family to know that he is having counselling. He says they wouldn't understand, nor, for that matter, would they stand for it. He is the family's support figure, and he has to be strong for them. He does not want to let them down. More than that, he sees himself as having to set an example. If he succeeds in life he will show them they can and will succeed themselves. If he has a good job, his brothers and sisters will be motivated to find a good job. It is working well for him. The training has shown him that he will enjoy the job. He stops and goes absent at a point when some of his family members are having difficulties. I talk to him about this. It looks like he is easing off the gas. We use the metaphor of the cycle racer at the front of the peloton. The rest are behind and wants to carry them in his wake. But if he starts going too fast for the others to keep up, he slows down and waits for them. They are his team mates. They are family. The, possibly unwritten, rule is that he won't ride ahead unless the others are with him.

This is his logic. Therefore the fact that he has stopped his training has nothing to do with the negative symptoms of an illness that determines the rest of his life. It has nothing to do with being unwilling or lazy. He has stopped training for the sake of family relationships. We explain this to the supervisors and he is not dropped from the scheme. He keeps his work placement. We are given time to talk about what has happened. It gives us points for discussion. How much of this family solidarity is down to choice? What does the solidarity entail? Are there other ways to show solidarity? Once he has considered this and talked it through, he is able to resume training.

Quartermaking is about explaining what went wrong with the colleagues who are trying to find him work, so they don't give up on him. His individual story, his relationship with his family, explains his apparently unfathomable and odd behaviour. The explanation opens up prospects for further work.

Discovering the relationship background as a way to understand a person's story and history, and having compassion for that, is much more humane and efficient than relying on classic diagnostics or a medical metaphor. This medical metaphor petrifies any prospect of a better future.

Explaining a client's odd behaviour to local residents by means of a diagnosis can be of help in gaining their understanding, but it can also lead them to feel pity for the person, who is then labelled as seriously ill. That person is still perceived as merely an object of pity and disappears as a person. Finding a personal logic to explain a person's odd behaviour and making that logic clear to the local resident is a greater guarantee of understanding without pity. It is a guarantee of compassion without losing that person to an illness, but letting them appear anew. It would seem that the telling of life stories is an extremely important part of this.

We search for people and places where people with mental ill health are welcomed as different. We search for niches, places where these differences can happily exist and are easily accepted. We search for techniques to keep the differences manageable and possible.

In the first part of this book, we talked about exclusion, which is often the lot of people with mental ill health. Historically, the social function of the psychiatric hospital has been to enable exclusion. It was a place to which people could be sent when they were no longer economically viable and created a nuisance.

Quartermakers prefer to organise hospitable places outside the mental healthcare setting, and so quartermaking is essentially the provision of hospitality outside the psychiatric hospital. Quartermakers try to improve niche diversity in society. The hospitable places are also described as niches. 'Niche' is a term used by Detlev Petry. A hospitable place has the following characteristics:

1   It is an environment with pleasing spatial proportions, people who are emotionally supportive with time to spare, and activities which the person in question sees as meaningful.
2   It is an environment in which the person in question is once again able to make his own choices, to see himself as an active person; has the

freedom to explore the value of his coping mechanisms (or survival strategies) for himself. An environment in which the person in question can develop a feel for his own worth; an environment open to co-ownership of the personal treatment process, as well as the organisation of which he is a part (Kal, 2001, pp. 67–68).

3 Another characteristic is the suspension of goal-resource-rationale. (…) It is not about making anything, producing anything, but about being present and together experiencing things that may be of value.

4 In a safe haven of this kind even the ideology of normality is suspended. There is space for otherness (Kal, 2001, p. 40).

It seems to me that the therapeutic community is an important place when developed along day-centre lines. The very fact that it is a day centre means that it cannot be a totalitarian institution that installs excessive dependence on the healthcare professional. As Tine Van Regenmortel says, we should be wary of the 'entrapping niche' (Rutenfrans-Stupar et al., 2019, pp. 329–348). An entrapping niche was intended as a home port, but also a base camp to society, but the second never materialised because 'ordinary spaces' were still inaccessible. Care professionals were not geared towards an accessible society, and professionals (and citizens) outside care were not geared towards people in the margins.

The practice of psychiatry is part of the social environment and in that sense it can also be considered a niche, a hospitable place for people with mental ill health. And this is a positive thing. Unfortunately, however, the medical model creates a situation in which the people that stay in the hospital can only identify with the role of the sick person, or the thing that no longer works. This is the sort of compassion that prevents people from developing and turns the hospitable place into a place of isolation. The concept of a mental disorder is nothing but a social construct. We do not wish to return to this anti-psychiatry idea. But we do hope that answers besides the medical model can be found for mental disorders. We hope for more niche diversity, and for niches in which people's vulnerabilities do not always have to be labelled as illnesses. People with mental ill health can only take up citizenship in a society that allows this variation of normality.

Treating someone who has been admitted to a psychiatric hospital means, first of all, sympathising with any feeling of exclusion they may have, with their feeling of being pushed to the side. It also means that, as a healthcare professional, you make every effort to undo that exclusion. A socially minded healthcare professional whose attitude to life gives him/her a sense of solidarity with people who find life difficult in society can be a basis for individual contact to blossom. As a healthcare professional, you question the structural aspect of the exclusion that is largely brought about by psychiatry. You as a healthcare professional are prepared to take social and political action to counter systemic exclusion. Community-based mental healthcare may offer a solution to this exclusion, provided the equality of the relationship between healthcare professional and patient is the key factor.

The danger with community-based care is that the classic medical model may also creep into the FACT teams, creating a sort of living room psychiatry, or psychiatrisation of society. I think that in Belgium Article 107 will have failed if we import the classical medical view from the psychiatric hospital to the FACT teams.

People who spend a long time in the psychiatric system face a whole of range of circumstances preventing their taking up of certain ordinary social roles. It is up to us, the healthcare professionals, to create new and better social conditions that give people more opportunities, and the courage to grasp those opportunities.

In essence, quartermaking is the organisation of hospitality (Kal, 2001, p. 57). It is being welcomed without question, unconditionally. Derrida talks about the foreigner who arrives in a country and does not speak the language (Derrida, 1998). There is a parallel here with the person who does not have a voice. We must ask ourselves whether that foreigner should know the language before s/he receives a welcome. S/he should not. Hospitality actually means allowing the foreigner to be a foreigner, and it means that s/he does not have to be like us before we accept her/him. From a philosophical viewpoint the word foreigner can have an objective connotation. There is a need to create spaces where this hospitality can exist, meeting places, room for difference.

One of the key words here is 'discord'. (free translation) 'There is talk of friction, of unease. There is something that just doesn't fit' (Kal, 2001, p. 174). The reason for emphasising this is that the idea is not for people with mental ill health to adjust to society. Paradoxically, the acceptance of difference is a precondition for integration. This acceptance of difference is also the acceptance of friction. Whereas assimilation and integration result in the unrealistic, utopian picture of peace, serenity and general well-being, quartermaking seeks to keep a more realistic model of tension and friction manageable for everyone. A social model that incorporates this friction is a society that knows that coexistence does not happen of its own accord and that the efforts needed to keep this coexistence possible are not exerted through the failure of this coexistence but are a necessary effort particular to coexistence itself. It comes down to finding or creating space for outsiders, and when these spaces are created, people are not forced to adapt to suit others' space. It is about finding places where meeting is possible, where oddness can continue to exist as oddness. And herein lies the paradox: odd is integrated as odd, and as different. This is discord. We can try to reduce this discord as healthcare professionals by speaking to local residents about mental ill health and about a person's individual mental health issues.

Quartermaking is too easily portrayed by its critics, and by cynics, as the process of finding a hospitable baker for a patient who is interested in baking bread. It is about much more than finding a specific place; quartermaking is not merely a dream factory that answers questions mechanically. You begin with a consideration of the patient's wishes, but stay alive to background and underlying questions relating to her/his past and the family circumstances. As a quartermaker, you try to get an insight into the very personal logic and dynamics of the person you are treating by (often literally) walking alongside that person in the hope of finding them a place that matches their story and history. It is a shared journey along which the quartermaker develops the talent to see or hear something that the client has not disclosed literally. It is being alive to the opportunity to discover a theme for the patient and recognise important pivotal moments in their treatment. It is together steering a path when obstacles appear; it is grieving the failures together and celebrating the successes together. In this sense, it is not a method but an intense meeting between people, full of empathy, compassion and understanding, and it is just as much about sharing insights, giving feedback and giving hope.

In her references to philosophers Doortje Kal mentions, as I have said, Luce Irigaray and the concept of wonder. She says that wonder can be a way to relate to others. Irigaray (1992) talks mostly about the difference of the sexes, but the idea can easily be applied to just about any other form of difference. Wonder precedes compassion, because wonder allows us to suspend the search for explanations. They are unnecessary. We allow things to stay incomprehensible. We refrain from the idea that we know the other, work on the basis that we do not, and allow ourselves to be surprised. Having a sense of wonder is an approach to life in which we resist putting people into boxes. Wonder is a way to approach others. It is often a quite a challenge to resist the urge to pigeon-hole: you have to suspend the idea of safety. Classifying a person creates a feeling of safety, because the classification can tell you how you should behave towards them. With wonder you take a risk. Suspending associations means suspending the feelings associated with them, such as the feeling of being unsafe. The idea of wonder can also be found in love. That beautiful feeling of being awestruck and transcending ourselves because we have discovered something we knew nothing about in someone else. Something strange that appeals to us. How much love is involved in being present with someone? The concept of 'love your neighbour' often draws on wonder. Being open to the unfamiliar. Opening yourself to the other, on the basis that you do not know them. It is also about letting go of the systems in which people are forced to function if they wish to meet.

The appreciation of art and beauty often rests on wonder. It fascinates us. We have the ability to set our knowledge and understanding aside. There is no need to compare what we are seeing, hearing or feeling with what we already know or recognise. We allow it to exist in its own right. This quality is strongest in outsider art (Roger Cardinal, 1972). A type of aesthetic that grips and amazes us because it cannot be taken in at a glance. The sheer amount of detail and repetition overwhelms us and places us outside ourselves.

4.5 Quartermaking Methods

Photovoice (Wang and Burris, 1997) is quite unique in that it can include a recovery element alongside a quartermaking element. Peer supporters, former patients and patients get together and select a photograph that reflects how they feel. There is also a worded caption, placed beside the photograph. The strength of the method lies in the combination of visual image and verbal caption. The group discusses the choice of photographs and texts, and they are presented as a whole, as a representation of this particular group. The presentation can then be given at an exhibition or in schools, community centres, etc. The technique was developed by Caroline Wang (university of Michigan) in the early 1990s (Wang and Burris, 1997). She conceived it as a creative approach to participatory action. It gives marginalised groups (people living in poverty, those with HIV/AIDS, (former) psychiatric patients, etc.) a voice with which to inspire empathy in others, and also to float ideas and so influence decision-makers. In other words, it is about generating more understanding, and, ultimately, improving the situation of the participants' community, but, most of all, it is about reducing exclusion.

Using community-based research activities, photovoice is a method designed to empower members of marginalised groups to work together to 'identify, represent and enhance their community through a specific photographic technique' (Wang and Burris 1997).

Multilogue (red. Heinz Mölders et al., 2017, pp. 81–102) sets up dialogue between clients, family members and friends. Healthcare professionals and people outside the mental healthcare setting are also included. Everyone is given equal status in the talks. The healthcare provider is not the person in charge at this meeting, but someone with a viewpoint to put to the others. The participants are no longer who they were after these talks, and, in particular (free translation) 'the client-relater has a free space where he or she, often for the first time, can relate his or her story and escape the monologue they had become trapped in' (Kal, 2001, p. 95).

Over the last two years I have had the privilege to chair seven meetings in Flemish cities with a view to setting up local quartermaking work groups. The local organiser invites a mix of people from mental healthcare and other sectors. Diversity among groups invited locally is high. This generates cross-border discussions between eight or so participants. Patients, ex-patients and family members often talk about the obstacles they face. It is very interesting to see meetings being attended by people in community development, as well as buddies and buddy coaches, the founders of halfway houses, etc. A colourful collection of people who share ideas and examine the obstacles and opportunities for integration. In one of the last meetings a former patient spoke about how hard is it for her, from the psychiatric hospital, to resume her maternal role for a child who has also been admitted to an institution. The meeting is attended by several people in KOPP projects (KOPP = Kinderen van ouders met psychiatrische problemen [Children of Parents with Psychiatric Problems]), who not only offer feedback but also gain new insights through the woman's story. These meetings are run in accordance with *multilogue* principles. Our experiment, a tour of Flanders, shows the vast potential for consultations of this type. By explaining the principles and positive results of quartermaking at one of these *multilogue* meetings, we are able to counter the sort of doomsaying and self-stigmatisation that leads to complaints with no traction. Most participants find the meeting extremely positive, and particularly encouraging in terms of generating more understanding and social space for people with mental ill health and their families.

Through *buddy projects* (Kal, 2001, p. 130), volunteers offer support on an equal footing to people as they emerge from social isolation (homosexual, lesbian, bisexual or transgender people, people with mental or psychiatric problems, people in poverty, refugees...) The support is often given in a one-to-one situation. An important aspect of this is doing things together, hanging out together. There are two processes here. One, is putting people in touch. Buddies are often volunteers who know very little about mental healthcare.

This aspect is important for some patients precisely because they already have plenty of contact with peers, and they need to be in touch with people outside the mental healthcare setting. But I would like to make the point again that quartermaking is not an ideology in the sense that all patients and former patients have to seek contact outside the mental healthcare setting. Some people focus on peer contact because it can enable more reciprocity than hanging out with a buddy. They find peer contact safer, closer to friendship, and the arrangements much less formal. Strictly speaking, then, peer contact is not quartermaking, but important nevertheless.

Secondly, volunteers can put the people they hang out with in touch with others. A type of organised friendship. And the main way of establishing contact is through presence. Selma Sevenhuijsen puts it like this:

> (free translation) Buddy services understand that people develop a sense of self and self-worth because there are others who acknowledge them and confirm their individuality, who attach value to their presence in the world and who make a very real effort to do justice to their capacities.
>
> (...) (free translation) Therefore buddy services could very well lead to the recovery of reciprocity.
>
> (Kal, 2012, p. 63, Sevenhuijsen 2000)

(free translation) The need to put on a public face is as basic as the need for the privacy in which to take it off. We need both a home that's not like a public space and a public space that's not like home.

(Franzen, 1998)

After years on a psychiatric ward people often become unused to being in public space. Sometimes, mired in self-stigmatisation, they can interpret the inability to connect as rejection. Public spaces, governed by certain social conventions that do not require personal exchange, are seen as hostile, no longer reassuring. Happily wandering is either mistakenly seen as an inability to connect or becomes so charged with negative meaning that the person feels unsafe. Going out with a buddy can help mediate this feeling. A buddy walks alongside you in the hope that public spaces can, once again, be a place to wander After all, it is by wandering carefree through public space that we become human again, and not just the carrier of an illness.

Going shopping together, to the cinema together, to the theatre, the zoo, the library, having a drink together with no need for any real personal or individual contact is what being out in public is about... This is because being human also involves contact through which we see each other, show each other that we are there, and no more than that. It is about making it possible to enter non-authoritarian spaces.

It is important to make sure that the person who asks for a buddy does not feel patronised or begin to feel dependent on the buddy. There is a danger that people with mental ill health, who may find it difficult to communicate, will begin to withdraw into isolation again. The presence approach can be of huge thematic value in this type of contact. When mentally ill people request a buddy they often do so because they lack a feeling of safety when in contact with others. The special thing about it is that they can be in a person's company without having to be on their guard. (free translation) 'At times it is (indeed) the other way round for the volunteer. He or she is aware of the insecurity that his or her buddy feels and tries to offer this security through his or her friendship' (Kal, 2001, pp. 146–147).

At times a volunteer may seek recognition from the person s/he goes out with and it is not given automatically. People with mental ill health may not always manage to express their satisfaction with or approval of this contact with the volunteer.

Where this reciprocity is impossible due to the mental health issues of the person who asked for a buddy, it is important that the buddy be able to get something back elsewhere.

I have the privilege to work with the people at *metawonen* in Ghent, a buddy project with many years of expertise. I have noticed that contact between buddies is extremely important. They express their appreciation of each other's efforts. It is also important that buddies receive frequent coaching and assistance from professionals. The buddy service is organised to ensure that the person assigned a buddy is matched with a buddy that suits him. Besides mutual interests, it is sometimes very important to be aware of the buddy's capacities when deciding who he can hang out with. If problems arise the coach can always intervene. This coaching role can also be filled by the professional who has the client in his care. It is he who knows the client well, and he, in liaison with the buddy-project coach, is best placed to establish communication between the buddy and the client or correct it if things go wrong. The professional can gradually move to the sidelines in his contact with the client by improving contact between the buddy and the client.

The 'IJsbreker voor een vreemde vogel' [ice-breaking] (Kal et al., 2012, p. 40) method sacrifices a part of the public space because the space itself is too threatening for the person with mental ill health or for others. A person with mental health issues would love to play badminton at a club, but knows that his behaviour under stress, such as compulsive thinking, hearing voices, etc., might ruin or disturb the public calm. The person with mental ill health cannot always observe the social conventions of the group. For that reason, one of the club's organisers is made aware of some of the person's traits. This person, often the club chairman, is aware of the new member's issues and can mediate with the other members should the need arise. The realisation that the club chairman is aware of the issues can give the new member a greater sense of safety and more confidence as a result. A very nice example of quartermaking is 'shared reading'. We have a similar initiative in the municipality.

A librarian, reads out the opening lines of a story about a boy who walks into a café early one morning. She leads the meeting in a little room above the library. And has laid on coffee and cakes. Three ladies from the municipality, along with Vera and Katelijne from the psychiatric centre, listen carefully. The room quietens as the librarian reads on. They all know each other. They have been to this meeting before. This time, the story is about a paper boy who comes in for a coffee after finishing his round. One of the customers has a story to tell the paper boy. The man talks about how, until he met the woman who would later become his wife, he had never had the opportunity for love. But the woman ran off with another man. The librarian stops reading briefly to listen to people's thoughts, feelings and ideas. They speak about loneliness and separation. Vera, a patient on our ward, listens and nods. When the librarian asks if anyone else would like to read, she volunteers. She starts hesitantly, before finding the right tone. The story assumes a more spiritual dimension when the man speaks of the peace he found five years after his divorce, and his discovery of science. Then it takes a strange turn and becomes difficult to interpret, hazier. People start talking again. The story is about love, but it is also about the illusiveness of the things that affect us, and about the things that bring us peace and the things that set us in motion. Vera feels the eyes of group upon her. They are calm and friendly eyes, so she talks about the things in life that have affected her. The story that she had been reading seems to encourage her to speak of her deepest motivations. Vera says that she is from a seaside town. That she will live in sheltered housing with others who have spent time on a psychiatric ward. She says that she has odd experiences sometimes. Vera feels entirely at ease with these people, who, by listening to this afternoon's story, have shown their respect for the intangible things in life, the incomprehensible things that needn't be frightening, but can actually be beautiful. She gets an encouraging and understanding response. They talk about the psychiatric centre, how the healthcare professionals treat the psychiatric patients. Katelijne, the escort, speaks about her work and how much she enjoys it. She talks about how the people who work at the centre, and stay there, are not affected by prejudice or negativity. She talks about the importance of the patients' strengths and vulnerabilities. The others at the meeting, the village residents, go on to discuss their own vulnerabilities. The librarian tells me about her 'Shared Reading' project.

> What it comes down to, perhaps, is that people in the psychiatric system (or from other more vulnerable groups) feel so comfortable at a "Shared Reading" group that they speak frankly with the others about what touches them in the writing, about how it connects to their own life. There is nearly always respect and mutual trust, because the climate places everyone on an equal footing. The leader-participant hierarchy does not exist. No one has a patent on the truth, everyone draws on their own abilities and understanding to interpret the writing. Vera attends several meetings and eventually begins to feel at ease, to the point where she begins to talk about her vulnerabilities. Other people say that they are touched by the beautiful things happening in psychiatry, by the way that people can be brought to a point where they see past the 'illness' and stop thinking that what they have here is a 'patient'.

> At a later meeting the librarian is there with four women from the community, Els, a nurse, and Jeroen, a patient from the ward. Els was a little worried that Jeroen would not show. But he was held up because his bike was stolen and he had to find another. This becomes the topic of conversation between him and the local residents. He keeps leaving the meeting for brief periods. He finds it very hard to keep his concentration and follow everything. His contact with other people can be quite flighty. He may suddenly leave the room in the middle of a conversation. On one such occasion he asks if anyone would like a coffee when he returns. The participants are very appreciative of the gesture. Anyone can read a passage from the day's story if they want to. Once again, the story prompts

a discussion and people share their personal experiences. A woman talks about her son, who is getting more serious about his judo, and Jeroen briefly responds by saying that he has done judo too, but had no choice in the matter. He tells the others that he doesn't know his nieces and nephews, and they find this strange. Then he goes on to read a passage from the story. The intensity of his reading and his beautiful intonation make quite an impression. Remarkably, now that he is reading, he keeps his concentration for a long time. The others are full of praise for his lovely voice. He has brought poetry, which he has written himself. Glancing at the stack of poetry, one of the ladies says that he must be very intelligent. Jeroen loves difficult words, which he mixes with newly coined words and phrases. He emphasises not the meaning, but the linguistic musicality. It is all about the sound. The poetry is like a spoken song. The lady listens, somewhat surprised. She is seeing and hearing something very special and says so. He sees her wonder and amazement and it does him good.

4.6 Quartermaking between Patient and Community

Walter is holding a bottle of whisky, wearing a helmet and stomping merrily around his neighbours' vegetable patches while making motorbike noises. For a long time now he has been talking about getting a car or a bike to go exploring with. He rattles the destinations off. It doesn't really matter, as long as he is on the move. In his rush to be off he has obviously overlooked his neighbours' vegetables.

Els, a fellow case manager on the ward, gets a call from Laura, Walter's next-door neighbour. Els attends immediately. Our psychiatric hospital is a ten-minute drive from Walter's home. She is greeted with the scene described above. Walter hands the whisky over, and Els has a word with the gathering crowd of neighbours.

We pay no attention to diagnoses. We believe in our clients' motivations, and we offer support when they run into obstacles. Talking things through with the neighbours is one way to help those who have been abandoned by others and detained in wards to get back on track.

The main thing bothering Walter's neighbours seems to be how safe it is to approach Walter when he does the sort of things described above. Walter is brought into the conversation. We tell him, in a friendly way, that this behaviour is out of order, and, in the process, we show the neighbours that Walter can be spoken to as they would any other neighbour who is up to something they do not like. Walter listens and agrees with Laura and the others.

Laura was the neighbour who got in touch about Walter. She was critical of our approach on behalf of the neighbours. She was reluctant when we initially asked if it would be okay for us to come and see her about Walter. She was afraid that we wanted her to babysit Walter. We reassured her, and we said that what we actually want to do is support the neighbourhood. She has our phone number, and we respond immediately when she calls. This way, Laura tells us of any concerns she may have about Walter.

She helps him. When she mows her lawn, she runs over Walter's lawn too. Her dogs run in and out of Walter's house, and he loves it. If she is there with him when we visit, we all have a coffee together. It is all very neighbourly. And the neighbours have come to know Walter too. They know his strengths and weaknesses, and they have found out that it is not dangerous to approach him. Laura is our permanent neighbourhood contact and mediator. For the time being, Walter is not allowed to sleep at home. We know that nights are the most difficult time, not so much for Walter but for the surrounding area, because there is no one to support the neighbourhood at present should anything happen at night.

He is going to the shops again for the first time since his psychosis, with us to escort him. Walter realises that we will do anything to help him realise his dream of a normal life. This makes him less impatient and aggressive when we tell him what he can and can't do. Stays on the locked ward are a thing of the past. Put simply, Walter is hopeful again, which means more and better communication between us and him and the neighbourhood he lives in.

Actually, we are a group of people who care for Walter, but not by absolving him of his responsibility for what he does or doesn't do.

Client, healthcare professional, parent or neighbour: it makes no difference. We are a group of people with a single goal, and that is to help a patient become a citizen again.

As for Walter's desire for speed and travel: while working towards a better and safer integration we found a neighbour who was prepared to take Walter for a ride on his motorcycle. This neighbour became our very first bike buddy.

Walter and others like him have shown that professionals are needed to exercise presence with the local residents. Their presence and commitment gives local residents the courage to speak out about their anxieties over Walter's unpredictability. The availability of the professional gives local residents a sense of safety, and this enables them to accept Walter in the community. The healthcare professionals are the ones who make it easier for them to understand Walter's behaviour. The better they understand it, the less unpredictable they will find him. Walter is fine with it. He gives a thumbs up to the people around him and adds that everything is okay. He obviously enjoys his neighbours' friendship. Only briefly mind, before he is off again. Happily cycling around the neighbourhood.

The local residents sometimes express their concerned but slightly stand-offish attitude to seriously abnormal behaviour with a smile and a shrug of the shoulders. This good-natured respect for difference is actually quite touching.

Quartermakers contact people outside their social bubble, their own reference group. Quartermakers support local residents, to keep them open to the idea of having a neighbour with mental ill health. In this sense, quartermakers are bridge builders.

> Marianne calls and asks me to come quickly, and she shows me a letter from the landlord giving notice on the rent. It says that she keeps a pet, and that this is not allowed under the tenancy. My client says that she suspects another reason. There had been a discussion a while ago with the upstairs neighbour, who rents from the same landlord, about the noise. The upstairs neighbour thought my client's CD was too loud. The local police were involved but the situation was never resolved. I ask my client if she minds me having a word with the neighbour upstairs. We have a relationship of trust, so she gives me permission to speak and negotiate on her behalf. I have a long talk with the lady upstairs. Well, not so much a discussion but a monologue from her. The fact that someone came to listen turned out to be very important. Her problems have become a lot worse in the meantime. She tells me that relations between her and my client were really good in the beginning, but that recently my client has been drinking alcohol, and, when she does, she cranks up the volume up on her schlager music. This talk with the upstairs neighbour gives me quite a lot of new information. What I hear is that my client feels lonelier than I had thought, which gives me information that will be of help to me in our conversations. I leave my card with the neighbour. She can call me and I will come at any time. We have established contact. I can mediate between her and my client.
>
> I accompany my client to the tenants' association to deal with the notice letter. The man there is matter of fact: you can't end a tenancy agreement because somebody buys a canary. He gives us a standard letter for the landlord and the matter is closed. I let the landlord know of our suspicion that the notice letter was motivated by a neighbouring woman's complaints, and I say that I am trying

to settle the matter between them. This tells the owner that we are taking the matter seriously and intend to resolve it.

The main thing I have learnt through my work with local residents who are having a problem of some kind with a mentally ill person, is not to be defensive, and to start by listening. There is no real need to say much in an initial talk with someone who has been building up resentment towards a client you are coaching over time. It is important to hear the reasons. What people remember most is the fact that you took the trouble to listen, and took the time to understand. The fact that you aim to take their problem seriously and would like to mediate is what allows you to rebuild that all-too-essential goodwill towards your client A good talk, a dialogue, is possible only when local residents have regained control over their anger and anxieties. At that point, you can give an explanation for your client's behaviour and thinking. You open the way to more empathy, and, through that, more understanding and compassion. If you talk it through with the client there is a good chance that s/he will be willing to cooperate after receiving some goodwill from the neighbours.

Another example. On reflection, Jacques experiences his psychotic episode as a break between who he was before the psychosis and who he is after it. The probation officer is of the opinion that he shouldn't speak about his psychotic episodes, as she thinks it could trigger the psychosis. I tell the probation officer that it is important for him to close the gap he feels in himself by actually talking about the psychosis. We practise quartermaking with the probation officer in order to bring a psychologist in. Jacques' psychotic experiences are very closely related to his faith, and for that reason we look for a priest who can give him voluntary work. He gets a job as verger. We do not run away from his psychotic experiences. At his asking we help with his search for the meaning of these experiences and manage to convince other significant people in his life to join in with this search for meaningfulness.

Another example. A client is served notice by the social housing agency. There have been occasional rows with the upstairs neighbour, and the rental office has noticed that the home is gradually beginning to get quite dirty. They add that it is not easy to get in touch with him and that he is unwilling to allow people in. We are told that it is best to catch him on a Monday morning, when he goes to draw money from the bank. I go to his home on a Monday morning and ring the doorbell. He gives me a rather fleeting and nervous look as I rush to explain who I work for. He pays me scant attention and says that he has to go to the bank. I ask if I can come along. He whispers something I don't catch and I take it as a 'yes'. He sets a blistering pace and I have to move quickly to keep up. He gives me the occasional glance. Conversation is not really possible. He goes shopping on the way home. I offer to help carry his bags. He agrees. We go back to his house together. I do this four times, and one day he invites me in for a coffee on our return. The home is indeed dirty. Old fruit and vegetable waste on the table and floor. I do a little tidying while we have our coffee, and he allows me to. He even seems to appreciate it. Over my next visits I notice a kind of manual awkwardness that prevents him from cleaning up. He attempts to wash a cup and gets so frustrated with all the fumbling around that he eventually tosses it in the bin. When I retrieve it and wash it for him he gives a satisfied nod and keeps saying the word 'example'. I assume he wants me to show him how to do it. Going out and about with him sets up a relationship of trust, and thanks to that we get an insight into why his home is becoming neglected. It becomes apparent that he knows his home is not as it should be, and that he is prepared to accept help with its upkeep. We now know that we can serve as a portal, through which the Family Care service can help him look after his home. We see ourselves as a liaison service. But first we need the Family Care service on board with the idea of home help. However, not all the conditions are satisfied. And this is where the quartermaking begins. How do we get the Family Care service to allow some flexibility in their procedures? We – a few of our FACT team colleagues and some people, mostly managers, from the Family Care service – meet with this question in mind. We remove a few of the obstacles that make him ineligible. He can barely put together a sentence, which means he is unable to complete the intake procedure. The man in charge of intakes agrees to let me and my colleague provide the information. The home is so dirty that the Family Care service would normally want it to be cleaned first. They are prepared to make an exception in this case. There is also the feeling that it might not be safe to clean his house. We agree that my colleague or I will be there in the first few months, when the Family Care people are in the house. At those times I ensure at least the minimum of communication. I have known the client for a while now and can pass on important information about what he does and doesn't like. We know that he appreciates the help. We have deduced this from his behaviour and can pass it on to the Family Care service. The Family Care people regard the collaboration as a kind of pilot project, an experiment, and both sides are proud of the result. It is enormously pleasing when people come to an accommodation over their organisation's rules and boundaries. You could call it quartermaking to organisations. As a quartermaker you encourage organisations to do something special for special people. It was also very gratifying to learn afterwards that, through their pride in this collaboration, the Family Care service has encouraged other, similar organisations to operate this way. If the clients themselves do not have the communication skills to express their satisfaction with the staff in other organisations, it is important that you send out messages and emails with the message that it couldn't have happened without their help. It is important to share your successes with organisations when you inspire them to be more hospitable. You get the feeling that together, very briefly, you made the world a better place. Over the years, by working in this way, I have developed a strong relationship of trust with organisations like the Family Care service. When I get in touch about a new client, they know to expect an exceptional request. And, on the strength of our dependable relations, they are always happy to entertain it. One of these new support services involved having a Family Care worker do three nights at a client's home to see if his restlessness was related to feeling lonely at night. This work yielded important information with which we were able to develop the client's home support.

It is important to be dependable in all your contacts with other organisations. The Family Care service workers are always given adequate details about a client's living circumstances and lifestyle. They are given the information they need to do their job to the best effect. The Family Care service understands that we are concerned about the safety of their staff. We are always ready and willing to provide support to their organisation if needed. In that sense we are always available to them. In all our endeavours we consider them equal partners, and we take their feedback and suggestions very seriously in the many meetings we have.

The most interesting thing is when we set up partnerships with organisations outside the mental healthcare setting. This enables patients to break free of mental healthcare services, and they are no longer patients or clients.

In Arnhem (the Netherlands), the Molendal hotel has set aside two rooms for people with mental ill health, to help them obtain rest. Clients pay ten euros a night towards the price of the room. The RIBW (a sheltered housing association) makes up the rest. It is known as the Bed & Break project. On arrival, guests are given a volunteer (sometimes a volunteer lived-experience expert) to go out with while staying at the hotel. Clients may use the room for no more than two weeks in any year. A quartermaking project, and one with no stigma attached. This is not some remote hotel set aside solely for people with mental ill health. The clients stay among the regular guests. Mental health issues or not, the staff treat every guest in the same way. This project is much less expensive than a ward admission, and much more comfortable for the client.

4.7 Quartermakers and "Meaningful Activity"

Healthcare professionals can get frustrated with patients who, against their better judgement, cling to activities which the former see as a waste of time.

> Karel has severe speech difficulties. A few words, not really in proper sentences. He is unable to complete activities without help. He lives independently in a small flat. He works with wood, constantly, but all his efforts fail. He wants to be a carpenter. Time and again, healthcare professionals have advised him not to look for work in this area, They do not think that he is up to it. Through contact with his family we learn that Karel's father is a carpenter. But his parents are no longer in touch with him. They see him as a failure in life. He is unable to talk about his parents. It seems that woodwork is Karel's way of seeking his father's approval. Woodwork is an unsuccessful attempt to narrow the gap between himself and a father who was bitterly disappointed at a son with mental disabilities. We do not advise Karel to stop his woodworking, but recognise the deeper meaning of this activity, and we work with him to find out how the bond with his parents can be restored.

Healthcare professionals try to combat inactivity or the so-called inactivity that goes with problem behaviours (drug misuse, hospital admissions, absconding, repeated requests for a locked ward...) by encouraging patients to take up a daily activity. The idea that many problems are avoidable by 'keeping occupied' is hardly a silly one. But it would be silly to impose it on clients as a means of solving those problems. For that matter, the mere coincidence of inactivity with problem behaviour does not imply a causal link.

And yet, not being there enough, or not allowing the suffering to be expressed, is often 'resolved' by viewing a patient's lack of activity as the main cause of the problem behaviour. This is when labels like 'taking advantage of the admission', 'laziness', or 'not ready for sheltered housing' crop up, on the assumption that the problem can be solved by activation.

When a person's behaviour seems incomprehensible or unfathomable and disturbing, and that person does not meet expectations, some professionals tend to see 'meaningful daily activity' as some sort of miracle cure. Being active, especially in a place where other health professionals can keep an eye on things, makes it look like the unfathomable will be contained. People assume they are promoting recovery by referring these people, against their will, to halfway houses or recreation experts who can point them to training centres or rehabilitation programmes. This lack of qualitative concern does nothing but reconvert patient time to organisation time. People assume they are supporting innovation in care by referring people to these new places, but this cannot be allowed to obscure the fact that the old relationship of 'the healthcare professional knows what is good for the patient' is raising its ugly head again. And then the patient gets the blame for anything that does not appear to work: 'You have these problems, and you are stuck with them, because of your inactivity'. In other words, it is the patient's fault. This attitude does not bother to untangle the knot of events that have led this man or woman into the situation. The danger of places like halfway houses, for example, is that they may end up being a sort of treatment referral service, and the referring coach has a list of facilities that offer resources for the patient to use. If the patient does not attend or refuses the offering s/he is deemed to be not engaged in meaningful activity. This treatment offering is also a product of the demand from other organisations (sheltered housing, probation).

Sometimes when people are taken away from conflict situations they become inactive in the place they are taken to. I have noticed that after an involuntary admission quite a few people eventually become inactive and indecisive about the direction of their life. Quite logically really. The direction they had wanted to take brought them into conflict with their environment and that was why they were taken away. The act of removing a person from their environment does not make them see the possibility of doing things differently after being admitted to a ward. It will often be necessary for the healthcare professional to return to the reason for the involuntary admission, to get an insight into the patient's current inactivity and the problem, which the admission does not automatically resolve.

If we make suffering expressible by understanding the logic behind it, we can offer tailor-made support, through which the healthcare professional's requirement of 'meaningful recreation' no longer applies and becomes superfluous.

> There is the man who is involuntarily admitted because he loves a person who does not wish to return that love. He cannot believe that the woman he loves so much does not want to start a relationship with him. The love remains and is still the main thing that motivates him. He can't get it out of his thoughts and appears unable or unwilling to engage with anything else. He has learnt not to talk about it, as nobody wants to hear. Eventually, the healthcare professionals forget what is on his mind, remembering only that he comes over as lazy and unwilling to do anything useful with his time.

It is the job of the healthcare professional to connect. This is where his or her relationship with the patient begins. You look for a meaningful daily activity only if the patient asks you to, and you do not use it to gain control over what you perceive as incomprehensible behaviour.

As a quartermaker, you get to work on any question that rises to the surface through being present with the patient, through listening to the tangle s/he is in.

On the subject of chronically ill patients, I believe that in the case of a chronic psychiatric issue it is no longer easy to tell whether, for example, the psychiatric problem, such as psychosis, was behind irresolvable financial, legal and professional problems or, conversely, these issues made the subject flee his desires and prevented him from finding the way back.

A flight from desires can be revealed through inactivity, passivity or the desire for medication, alcohol or obliterating drugs. The patient has already tried to escape his/her difficult and often hopeless situation many times, and it has always led to a crisis, so s/he stops trying. The advantage of calling it 'a flight from desires' is that we can assume a desire still exists, and, as healthcare professionals we have to work on this assumption. This is the challenge when working with patients who are or were in for a long stay.

You work with them to untangle the knot. This process of working together to find an activity with meaning for the patient is described beautifully in individual placement and support (IPS) (Drake et al., 1999, pp. 289–301). When looking for a job the counsellor ties to connect with the client's desires or wishes. This approach is diametrically opposed to the offer of courses or training to raise people to a higher level. The training and coaching is given not in preparation for the job, but in the place where the job is carried out.

> On one of her visits to the Netherlands a colleague of mine hears a counsellor talk about a very confused man whose only wish is be an aircraft pilot. She takes his wish very seriously and tells him that she will look into it with him. They drive to Schiphol several times and wander around the airport, striking up conversations with people. The IPS counsellor soon sees that the man is very attentive to the stewardesses there. He waves at them, and it does him a lot of good when they wave back. The IPS counsellor helps him get a job with the airport cleaning crew. In this job he gets to see 'his air hostesses' pass by every day, and it makes him really happy. IPS is quartermaking in the sense of helping a person find a daily activity or job. It is about looking at what the patient wants, and not the healthcare professional's desire to get someone to be more active and thereby control what the healthcare provider sees as problem behaviour.
>
> In the example I used to introduce the chapters on recovery and quartermaking we saw how people became active through the feeling of having meaning for someone. Quartermaking is about finding places in which these people can do something for someone else. It is about finding or creating places where reciprocity is made

possible again. We saw that the couple's desires related to activities in which they were once successful. She wanted to find a good home for the branded clothing she wore as a business manager, and he, a former chef, wished to help create meals for local residents. This enabled them to restore a little of their pride and helped to heal the break with the life they had once led.

It is up to the healthcare professional to join the client on the journey to a hospitable place that suits the client. Once the connection has been established, the next and final stage is to extend it, mostly by supporting carers, volunteers, peer supporters, employers and others in the network. You view the people in the network as expert and competent and trust them to support your client. Above all, you set out to empower these carers and family members. In the best circumstances you will make yourself, as a healthcare provider, surplus to requirements, and you will remain available in case the network needs to draw on you in the future.

4.8 On Outsider Art and Quartermaking

Might outsider art (Roger Cardinal, 1972) be a niche for people with mental ill health? Does this niche keep the practitioners of outsider art on the margins of society? Or is outsider art a style that exists independently of the artist's social standing? And what about community art? Art is the best way for us to experience what we do not know, what is alien to us, and it can be extremely beautiful and absorbing.

His door is always ajar. The people passing in the corridor make him feel less lonely. I pop in every day. Others do too. He is a calm and amiable man, with short hair and a grey beard. Fons has converted his tiny room in the psychiatric department into a studio. The easel stands in the centre of the room. The bed is in the corner. Coloured splashes of paint are collecting on the floor and the wall. Even his palette is an abstract masterpiece, and it gets more beautiful with every painting. Oils, nothing but oils. He thinks acrylics are for amateurs. Art books on the shelf. There is always jazz in the background, Charles Mingus preferably, the double bass player and composer. Fons proudly shows me the glowing liner notes on the LP *The Black Saint and the Sinner Lady*. The text was written by Charles Mingus's psychiatrist. Their relationship went from doctor/patient to fan/artist. And that describes my relationship with Fons. I see him as an artist more than a patient.

In one way or another his works are comforting and hopeful, even the ones on the concentration camps. He has a portrait of himself between his parents: a black and white drawing. Only his wide-open mouth is a deep red, to express the pain. A blazing colour like a silent scream.

He has portrayed himself in a hospital bed. No hands, just stumps, and a face contorted in pain. Above his head a maze of lines that appear to symbolise the disorder and chaos in his mind, caused by the many voices he was hearing. Fons never explains his paintings in much detail. He calls them 'little pictures' in his West Flanders dialect, as if they are worthless trifles. He finds it important for people to like his work. It encourages him to paint more. For a psychiatrist with children he paints a child playing on the beach by the sea. Same style, but entirely different content. Much cheerier.

Over the years I have met several inpatients who have created extremely interesting paintings and special drawings. On the ward we always allow them to work in the best circumstances possible. Talent should always be given the opportunity to develop. We contact museums and specialist galleries to recommend their work. We ourselves arrange regular group exhibitions at which patients are given the opportunity to show their work to a wider audience.

She walks into the big room with the long table looking straight ahead. People do not seem to interest her. The tables and the chairs: she knows them better than anyone else, stand where they have always stood when she has visited this studio over the years. As always, she sits in the space by the window, dips the brush in the water and then first in the pot of yellow paint. Someone has set everything out for her, so she can come and work with clockwork regularity. She does what she always has done, and it looks like she doesn't even have to think. She applies paint to paper and produces the colourful fairytale scene that appears to be stored in her mind. She tells me the story of her father, who was a space traveller. She writes letters to children who do not exist. I watch on, and at that moment I realise that something very special is happening here, and that this story and this woman's actions, her painting, will change my life. It is the late1980s, and I am on placement at the psychiatric hospital. I hear about 'outsider art' and 'art brut' for the first time. For the first time I see the often very colourful and quite busy, intense and highly detailed painting, sculpture, pottery and needlework. I am overwhelmed, but above all fascinated. It is the creative therapist and artist Jacques Ponceau who tells me about the people who work, day in, day out, in his studio. Jacques will become a very good friend. For the patients who came to his studio he was more companion/artist than a healthcare practitioner, and, above all, he provided the paper, paints and other materials with which these people went to work so intensely. Each had a distinctive style. I remember the TV report about Jacques' trip with his artists to the museum of modern art. They weren't very impressed with the art, because they felt there wasn't enough craft in what they saw there. I was extremely sympathetic to their very honest and matter-of-fact view. But they didn't talk their own work up, or even have very much to say about it. They found it quite annoying to have to stop and talk about their work. They just wanted to carry on. I remember a woman who embroidered the edge of her embroidery, to frame the piece. Jacques had to take it out of her hands, literally, because the frame was getting bigger and broader. When given a new piece of material she simply started a new piece of embroidery. She didn't really look at what she had produced. The act of making it was more important than the product.

There are several ways of looking at artworks produced by psychiatric patients. The first is the diagnostic view. This rests on the belief that the bond between mind and artistic expression is so strong that a change in one initiates a corresponding change in the other (Berge, 2000, p. 78). The best example of this view relates to the work of Louis Wain (1860–1939). Most of his paintings and drawings were of cats. He was diagnosed with schizophrenia. Psychiatrists place his quite diverse works on a timeline, where the more abstract pieces corresponded with his growing symptoms of schizophrenia. In other words, the absence of a figurative aspect was said to reflect the worsening of his symptoms. It turned out that the psychiatrists had manipulated the timeline to lend credence to their theory (Berge, 2000, p. 80). In actual fact, Wain also did figurative paintings at times when he was at his most psychotic. From the diagnostic viewpoint, art is described as 'psychotic art' and 'schizophrenic art'. The artists shown by example are not mentioned by name because their work is seen as the outcome of a disease rather the outcome of an individual's work. A painting reflects the damage to the brain caused by psychosis and is no longer the work of an individual.

It is a view that gives early psychiatry a means by which to be taken seriously as a new science. The creative forms of expression are seen as a diagnostic tool to tell us something about a person's mental state. Changes in the style or form of the subject indicate changes in the illness. (free translation) 'This comes through making the mistake of not seeing the romantic pursuit of genuine self-expression as a relatively new ideal in some artists, but as a definition of art in general' (Berge, 2000, p. 78).

In the end, modern art was seen as the result of an (undesirable) departure, and this view reached its peak in the 'Entartete Kunst' exhibition arranged by the Nazis in Munich in 1937 (Berge, 2000, p. 81). An exhibition which then toured 11 cities in Germany and Austria with works by cubists, impressionists, expressionists, dadaists, etc. Many of these 'degenerate' art works were auctioned off at well below their market value. The leftover works were stacked and – like the un-German books before them – burnt in the barracks of the main fire station in Berlin. The auction revenue was used to expand the 'real German art' collections of various museums. Whereas they began by examining the art of psychiatric inpatients for characteristics that were symptomatic of their illness, they now saw art that generally differed from figurative works as indicative of a mental illness, and this sort of illness was thought to characterise the degenerate, the inferior person who was deserving of euthanasia or simply death.

In the diary of Hannah Höch, under Saturday 11 September 1937, we find the following text.

> The most important works from the postwar years are here. All the museums and public collections are represented here. After the public persecution it's astonishing how disciplined the audience is. There are a lot of closed faces and you can see opposition in many of them. Barely a word is said.
>
> (Höch, 1937, p. 585)

The diagnostic view has almost entirely disappeared now. I see it now and again when an artist's drawings are used to show how his/her mind is affected by dementia. A sort of final stage is also shown, in which drawn faces are no longer recognisable as faces.

The departure from the diagnostic discourse is initiated by a number of psychiatrists. Paul Gaston Meunier, under the pseudonym Marcel Réja, wrote *L'Art chez les fous* (1907), Prinzhorn wrote *Bildnerei der Geisteskranken* (1922) and Walther Morgenthaler wrote *Ein Geisteskranker als Künstler* (1921), about Adolf Wölfli.

By Morgenthaler and several other psychiatrists, the person with mental ill health was considered an artist for the first time, and style diagnostics were abandoned. But this new turn carried other risks for thinking on psychiatry, mental ill health and art.

> (free translation) Yet in more than one case we see that even in the psychological context the "style diagnostic" involves a not inconsiderable risk of unjustified psychologisation and marginalisation. When in the 20s the diagnostic dialogue began to make way for artistic appreciation the pathologisation came to an end. But the ensuing glorification of outsidership did not bring an end to marginalisation.
>
> (Berge, 2000, p. 83)

In Prinzhorn, in particular, we see this idealisation of the outsider emerge for the first time. Prinzhorn was highly sympathetic towards the expressionists and only too pleased to support and confirm their take on art, which he appeared very well placed to do through his profession. The expressionists saw (free translation) 'the artist as an unworldly genius that derived his powers of creation from an inspired urge to create rather than education and application' (Ibid., p. 83).

Prinzhorn spoke of an original *Gestaltungsdrang*, or creative urge, which is present in all people but can be lost with the development of civilisation. He professed that mental patients who had long been isolated from society through confinement rediscovered something of that original creative urge. Psychosis would free up certain mental processes, though which this art would be produced. Psychosis and social isolation were therefore the reason behind the authenticity and originality of these people's work. However, his correspondence with the institutions revealed that it was he who gave the patients their materials, and that he paid them to paint, and so it was he who created the outside stimulus which he so vehemently denied.

(free translation) By presenting their mental and social isolation as the preconditions for their purity, he also contributed unwittingly to their further, symbolic removal from society. Only at a respectable distance could the mentally ill person serve as the Rorschach blot onto which insiders such as him and the expressionists, and later the surrealists, could project their ideals. Just like the non-Western primitive, the lunatic could be worked loose from every social, cultural and psychological context, and served up as an example of freedom and purity that could rejuvenate the art and culture.

(Ibid., p. 84)

Jean Dubuffet first spoke of 'art brut' in the 1940s. By this, he meant a group of ordinary people, selected by him, who created works far removed from art courses and art markets. He stressed the spontaneity of these art creators, their lack of schooling and a purity that came mostly from their isolation. When it turned out that some of his potential selectees were actually trained in the arts, or at least corresponded with art circles, he created the new category of 'Neuve Invention' for them, thereby creating a new class of artist, which he considered as less pure than those of art brut.

It became more apparent, however, that this purity was an illusion and that everyone is influenced by the culture they belong to. Wölfli (1864–1930), a Swiss artist who was one of the first to be associated with Art Brut, was aware of Swiss folk art, made collages from the magazines at his disposal and, as described above, knew of the interest in his work, of an audience, and so created works to sell – which Morgenthaler called 'bread art'. In the end, Dubuffet saw 'art brut' as an ideal to be aspired to, rather than a reality.

Michel Thévoz, Dubuffet's successor as director of the Collection de l'art brut in Lausanne, took the ideal so seriously that he lamented innovations in psychiatric care such as social integration. He thought that isolation was a necessary precondition for patients to produce art brut and was against allowing magazines and televisions into institutions where patients produced drawings and paintings (Berge, 2000, p. 86). He was not keen on the idea of studios for patients, because he thought that the originality of the work was influenced by the therapist's presence. Nor was he keen on medication to reduce the symptoms of psychosis, for he believed that it was the psychosis that gave the work its originality. At the very least you might question the ethics of anyone who argues against providing care or improving a person's health for the sake of the art they produce.

Thévoz's propositions are open to criticism, as is his view of the relationship between art and illness, and between art and environment. May art brut artists take elements from their environment as inspiration for what they produce and use the material without compromising their own style, as seen in the example of Willem Van Genk's work (Ans van Berkum, 1998). Studios for people with mental ill health or mental disabilities are very respectful of the guest artists' works. The offer of new or different materials often opens paths that the artists would not otherwise take. Ethics aside, the use of medication in general, such as neuroleptics, can affect a person's activity by shutting it down, but, given in the right dose, can just as easily allow them to avoid periods of crisis and so maintain their creativity.

April 2010. I meet Daniel Johnston backstage at the Ancienne Belgique concert Hall in Brussels. He achieved world fame in the 1980s when MTV picked up on his cassette-taped music. He has bipolar disorder, but, despite this, makes some very original music. His success reached a peak when Nirvana's Kurt Cobain wore a tee-shirt bearing his name and the name of his album. Johnston goes on tour but experiences frequent psychotic crises and is admitted to psychiatric institutions on several occasions. Medication, more than anything else, is what brings stability. When I meet him he is pretty friendly, and he tells me about his work. I am hugely impressed after our meeting, as I can see how much effort it takes for him to concentrate. On stage, I see a man who is clearly suffering with the side effects of his medication, such as weight gain and shaking hands. We might also assume that he has diabetes. Performing is extremely important to him. The treatment seems to be all about enabling him to continue his favourite activity. He accepts the medication as a part of this. Johnston also has a gift for drawing. His works are very popular. *The devil and Daniel Johnston* (Feuerzeig and Rosenthal, 2005) is a moving documentary of his life and creativity. As I see it, he is one of those people who, despite his vulnerability, and by revealing his vulnerability, succeeds in developing his talents and building a very meaningful life. I cherish the drawing he made for me and the photograph of us sitting together.

People like Daniel Johnston are able to perform again by taking neuroleptics. But suppose a person would rather experience quality of life without art than a nightmare existence, producing amazing artworks. Wouldn't we want them to enjoy the former? No one has the right, no matter how brilliant the artwork, to demand that its creator live in permanent distress to keep the works coming. There are a number of ethical questions to consider. The things said or produced by the creator are not always intended as art. It is often another artist who draws attention to the exceptional qualities of the outsider's work and discovers the outsider-artist in the process.

Adolf Wölfli found a good solution to the problem of his sudden artistic recognition and need to continue his mission by creating little paintings which he would sell to others, among them health professionals. This was his 'bread art'. He used the money to buy materials to draw and paint his oeuvre, which was based on the mission attached to his psychotic experiences.

We, and the artist, gain a clearer understanding of outsider art if we define it on the basis of style rather than the artist's social standing.

> When I mentioned outsider art to Fons, and wanted to present him as an outsider artist at the opening of his exhibition, he wasn't happy with the idea. He was a man of few words, but made it quite clear to me that he was an ordinary artist and not an outsider artist. He did not wish to be part of a group that lay outside the artistic mainstream or produced art on the fringes. He had a deep respect for people like Rik Wouters and emulated them. He wished to be counted among them, not in a group of psychiatric patients who practised art. It was the art that allowed him to rise above the identity of patient. He was an artist in a psychiatric hospital, not an excluded person who made art in an effort to belong. He wanted to be judged on the quality of his work. He wanted me not to be too emphatic either about his work for the ward magazine. It had too much of a therapeutic ring about it, which made him feel like a patient. He thought of it as a pastime, and as a gift to us. His paintings were his real work.

The term 'outsider artist' may seem to tie in with the idea of quartermaking by allowing a person to connect with the art world, but it could actually give them a sense of being labelled as something or someone they do not want to be, and that is an 'outsider'. Here I would argue that not all patients who draw and paint are outsider artists. I would argue, in a general sense, that the quartermaker should operate on a person's behalf within the conditions set by that person. That person cannot make an informed decision unless you have given a clear explanation of your method and how it is likely to affect him/her. If you intend to relate a work to an outsider collection it is important that its creator wishes to be defined in that way. It is also important to discuss how a person sees himself, and to have respect for that. If we romanticise marginalisation, there is a very real risk of leaving the people stranded there. The healthcare professional's desire to liberate a person from the identity of patient by applying the 'outsider artist' label will soon become dogmatic if there is no acknowledgement of the permanently shifting logic of the situation, or, especially, if it is contrary to the patient's feelings or wishes.

> (free translation) Outsiderism implies the preservation of outsidership, not, as in the diagnostic discourse, through a process of pathologisation, but through a process of marginalisation, where those concerned are more or less artificially kept at a distance so as not to endanger their status as archetypal Other and not to have to waken from the comforting dream of a last reserve of innocence and purity.
>
> (Berge, 2000, p. 90)

Outsider art is not the exclusive preserve of people with mental ill health, nor is it the exclusive preserve of people who live on society's fringes. People with mental ill health, whether on the fringes of society or not, can create outsider art or ordinary art.

In recent times, I have met many people with mental ill health who have professed to create art and for the sake of convenience have chosen to categorise their work as outsider art. They believe that their exclusion gives them the right to label everything they produce as outsider art. The quartermakers' idea that outsider art offers a niche for safe creation through which they can find a place in the community is good to begin with, but to say that anyone who is socially excluded and creates a piece of work is an artist by virtue of the fact that they are an outsider, is an injustice to art. It often reduces the concept of outsider art to a hobby and the product of creative activities. Adhering to the characteristics of style described above as a means to assess outsider art allows for an appropriate appreciation of the quality of the work.

James Brett (Museum of Everything) went for a different perspective when criticising the idea that 'outsider art' and 'being outside art' are equivalent terms. His touring museum exhibits quite a few works by people who are usually labelled as outsider artists. In October 2016, he founded the 'Gallery of Everything' in London. And as he wanted to avoid that particular categorisation of this art form he decided to dispense with the term 'outsider art' altogether. The artists who create outsider art are no different from ordinary artists and do not need a separate term:

(free translation) All of that conceptual jargon that they love so much in modern art comes down to the same thing. Art is a way of finding your own place in the world. You see that there (in the exhibition of the Museum of Everything).

(Steve Dow, 2017)

James Brett was intrigued by the name 'Museum of Everything' when he saw a photograph in the paper of the 80-year-old William Brett, unrelated, in a room full of the objects he had collected. The caption to the photograph read 'William Brett in the museum of everything'. The man is a local celebrity on the Isle of Wight in the UK. His house had been given that name by the local children. To James Brett it seemed like the ideal name to escape the term outsider art, which he disliked so much: (free translation) 'it reduces the art only to what it is not, thereby confirming the idea that this art does not belong to the artistic sphere' (Brett, 2016). The nice thing is that he dispenses with a term that emphasises the outsiderism of this art form, but it is a shame, on the other hand, that an art form, which does have specific characteristics, independent of the position and biography of the artist, can no longer be described in that way.

Let us plead for a new term that does not refer to the things going on in the margin of the arts (when relinquishing its status as a gallery the current museum in Brussels changed its name from 'Art en marge' to 'Art et Marge'). One solution might be to return to the term 'art brut', but without the connotations that Dubuffet and Thévoz introduced in relation to the art brut artists.

When we organise an exhibition through the psychiatric hospital in the municipality in 2015, it is not conceived as 'art by psychiatric patients' but as an exhibition in which everyone, including local residents, patients and staff, is free to participate. We do not want to highlight the difference between the participants by labelling them as patients, local residents or members of staff. The exhibition is set up in a space above the library in the municipality, a public space in the village itself, where we wish to integrate. The exhibition is conceived as a meeting place, as a way to allow those who are excluded and isolated to re-emerge from their isolation. The mayor's opening speech emphasises this. In his eyes, the patients are local residents. The pieces exhibited are a way of showing that what the patients paint and draw and how they do it are not unlike the local residents. It is an exhibition that gives 'amateur artists' the opportunity to show their work. Expressing yourself through art is a way to invite empathy and interest for many people in isolation. We always do this in collaboration with people who have nothing to do with psychiatry. Local residents exhibit works and help with the organisation. The opening reception is also organised by local residents and patients. Through *Kiosk* we would like to aim for more integration and less segregation in several ways.

This ties in with what is known as community art

> (free translation) in which professionally schooled artists work intensively with people who, normally, would never or hardly ever come into contact with active artistic practice. (...) Artists see people in their neighbourhood growing apart. They decide to bring people together and to think up an activity, which may even be to counter the degradation. For that reason they go out into the neighbourhood to see what can be done.
>
> (Kal, 2001, p. 16)

A work of art by a deceased outsider artist can be a meeting place for community building. We see this in Watts (Los Angeles). There, between 1921 and 1954 an Italian immigrant, Simon Rodia (1879–1965), created two towers with his own hands. They consist of 17 connected sculptures. The tallest tower is 13 metres high. The majority of the structure is made from recycled materials, such as bottles, shells, mirrors... He built it all with his own hands. Children and adults brought empty drinks bottles to be built into the tower. He himself would scour the area by foot for waste materials within a radius of 30 kilometres from the construction site. He left the structure to a neighbour in 1955. He had grown tired of fighting the authorities for planning permission. He moved to his sister's in Martinez (California) and would die ten years later without ever returning to Watts. The building was to be demolished in 1959. But there were protests. Its continued existence would depend on a safety test. A crane pulled on the towers, but it was the crane that broke down in the end. The foundation of the towers would set a pattern for other buildings. To this day, the towers are considered as Southern California's most culturally significant site. The Watts Towers Arts Center was built on the site in 1970. In 'Building Community Through Self-awareness and Self-expression', Gail Brown (2015, p. 327) describes how she gives a photography workshop at the location: 'From Where I'm Standing photo-documentary', in which local residents create photo documentaries with captions about their own lives: (free translation) 'Young and old work together and independently of each other in a supportive community environment. We go in search of their core values, their identity in supportive community environment. They also show their concern for the world around them'.

Participants are given the use of a camera for several weeks to take photographs, write texts and create a folder for exhibition. The Watts towers are often depicted as a monument to be proud of, colourful and creative, made by an ordinary person who exceeded himself through this creation. Some of the beauty of this place and its creator shines on the life and dreams of the people who live here, and it is accentuated by exhibiting these folders at the location.

Children and adults in Watts have a need and desire for something they can identify with other than the poverty and violence that surrounds them; from themselves and others they need recognition as the heroes – heroes in the sense of Joseph Campbell – they actually are, as people who create beauty and meaning from the raw materials in their life. There is a resonance between the workshop, the Arts Center and Simon Rodin's Watts Towers.

(Ibidem, p. 336)

More of these outsider sites around the world seem to be taking on a social function and contributing to community building. Outsider work in all its simplicity and fascinating magnitude gives inspiration and creates connections.

On the grounds of La Fabuloserie (Dicy, France), among works by many other outsider artists, I got to see the Pierre Avezard's life work (1909–1992), his 'Le Manège de Petit Pierre'. He used waste materials to construct a miniature world of towers, airplanes, trains, cows. A motor attached to belts of all kinds brings the whole piece rattling to life, and the little figures turn around. It must have been a gargantuan task to put it all together and it has resulted in something really naive and touching, but, through its sheer size, quite overwhelming. You do not know what to look at first. Avezard and his farm were famous before his piece was transferred to this outdoor, outsider collection in Dicy, and he would get many visitors, mostly children, on a Sunday. He had managed to build a real museum of his own.

Avezard suffered from Treacher Collins syndrome, a hereditary disorder of the head, which left him facially deformed and mute. For that reason he lived a very isolated life. The creator portrays himself in several places in the work. In one, he is a tiny figure dancing with his favourite cow. The deformity left him unable to find a dance partner, let alone a relationship partner.

The beauty and emotion of 'Le Manège de Petit Pierre', but above all the sophistication and persistence needed to create it are good portals to the social exclusion the creator experienced and how he managed to overcome it through his work. Schoolchildren are often brought to this place. The story of Petit Pierre gives children an insight into the importance of respecting people that look different or behave a little oddly. In other words, the work of an outsider artist who lived in social isolation is being used here as teaching aid to counter exclusion. Creation and art can be used in any number of ways to produce social exclusion. As long as 'outsider artist' does not refer to a particular style, it would appear that, by calling themselves outsider artists, painters and sculptors with mental ill heath can identify with a label that points merely to social exclusion. But then again, mental ill health and exclusion seem to lead to reconnection through art. It is by uncoupling the words art and exclusion that we avoid an 'us and them' situation, where we have artists on the one side and artists with mental ill health on the other. If we wanted to maintain this classification we could just as easily concoct names for artists with kidney diseases or pulmonary disorders, as a way to gain recognition for people with these illnesses. So it seems that by doing this we would set up a new diagnostic discourse designed for a positive discriminatory effect. Quite a few of the people who produce art and suffer from mental ill health feel belittled by this type of recognition, as it comes solely by way of their mental ill health and not on the strength of their work.

It is extremely important in my view to keep a term that continues to describe the 'art brut' style, only without the connotations added by Dubuffet and Thévoz. Whether coincidental or not, many art brut artists have mental health issues.

I would say that a very interesting route to connection and inclusion for people with mental ill health, in terms of quartermaking, is the process of creating 'community art'. Collaboration on a group outcome where artists and other people, patients, local residents... take part on an equal footing. This is because spending a long time on a project and bringing it to a satisfactory conclusion can eliminate many of the prejudices towards people with mental ill health.

4.9 More Social Solidarity

Care provision' is not literally bound to 'caring', but is primarily located in the provision of facilities in aid of citizens' social and cultural lives.

– Marius Nuy, *De nacht van Nederland*, 2001, p. 62

In quartermaking, we start with the patient who has become citizen again, whom we guide towards life in society and cooperation with other citizens. But we might also start with society. We assume that a differently organised, more hospitable society, could make quartermaking easier from the individual perspective, or even superfluous in an ideal world.

(free translation) Quartermaking should counterbalance a culture of commoditisation, monetisation (economisation) and objectification, because people with a psychiatric background do not thrive is this kind of climate.

(Kal, 2001, p. 38)

Primary prevention aims to prevent people from getting into serious psychological trouble. Tertiary prevention aims to improve the quality of life for people with a chronic psychiatric problem'. It is my belief that tertiary and primary prevention touch each other or form part of a circle. The better society is for chronic psychiatric patients, the better it will be for people who are vulnerable, for one reason or another, to psychiatric problems.

(Ibid., p. 39)

Could we reorientate society to define the concept of 'normality' differently? Could this type of society alter in moments of crisis? Aaron Hurst (2014) talks about major disasters that inspire us to courage, resourcefulness and innovation, and how they force us to redefine the concept of normality.

But this society, which allows the former patients, the new citizens, to find their place among the others... what would it look like? What sort of society would allow this connection to happen easily? How would rehabilitation or restoration to honour take place? By 'restoration of honour' we mean former patients being able to rediscover their place in society. In what model would these people's issues be accepted?

The challenge lies in the creation of citizenship that makes room for inclusion. If, through change and innovation, we can develop structures that influence relations between people, in the sense of less social inequality and exclusion, an influence will also be exerted on what we call 'normal'.

If hard times and crises in people's lives are the very time to introduce reform, then, by analogy, economic crisis is the very time for alternative social developments.

The idea of the *suspended coffee* is that a customer voluntarily buys a coffee not just for her/himself, but for someone unknown to her/him who comes along later. The second person asks for this 'coffee in waiting'. This practice is best known in Naples, as the *caffè sospeso*, and it took off in our country too in recent years. Since then we have also seen the phenomena of the suspended soup, suspended French fries, suspended fish fry, suspended haircut, etc. In Flanders the non-profit *Enchanté* organises hospitality from tradesmen. It is modelled on the Parisian organisation *Le Carillon*. One of the negatives is that these projects do not actually lead to more social contact between giver and receiver, so it is difficult to create the potential for reciprocity, where the receiver gives something in return.

In the chapter on recovery, we talked about reciprocity and how it relates to citizenship. We saw how reciprocity can be pursued in the relationship between the healthcare professional and the patient. How do we see the element of reciprocity in quartermaking?

If we take participation to mean a duty to take part in society, through compulsory volunteer work if needs be, or penalising people who do not take part, then this is not what we mean by quartermaking.

Quartermakers see people who are incapable of reciprocity as a result of their disabilities as people who have not been given enough opportunity to develop in a society that has not been hospitable enough.

In the Netherlands we see politicians, under what they themselves refer to as the 'participation society', attempting to organise that reciprocity by cutting services, in the idea that citizens will adopt these tasks with greater spontaneity and willingness.

When people are in receipt of a benefit they are expected to do something in return. This is known as 'the consideration'. In Rotterdam, for example, people are expected to go out onto the streets with litter pickers in exchange for their benefits. This sort of reciprocity causes resentment in people who have often worked for quite a while before becoming unemployed and, through the taxes they have paid, have already built up an entitlement to benefits. And the work they are required to do in return for their benefits is not in any way related to their education. They often experience the whole thing as a humiliation. It is clear that this kind of participation society simply pushes people further into poverty. This is because when the benefits are taken away people do not suddenly return to work.

Citizens need to care for each other more, and to achieve this we cut back on services.

Citizens are also increasingly expected to manage libraries, playgrounds and community centres, to keep their streets and neighbourhoods tidy, to keep criminals at bay, operate a shared community helpline, support each other through mental crisis and much more. In the 'care setting', the change goes far beyond simply offering more help at home. We already have care units where relatives are required to run 'voluntary' services. Compulsory volunteer work was once an oxymoron, but now it is a standard component of this revolution. To accommodate these staff cutbacks, it is entirely 'logical' to have people volunteer for 'downgraded employment'. In quite a few municipalities, 'volunteer work' is now compulsory for benefit recipients, immigrants and others claiming state assistance. The new motto is that if you get something, you should give something in return.

For part of their lives, or even the rest of their lives, many people with mental ill health are not in a position to reciprocate. Quartermakers act on their desire for reciprocation, and not on the state's desire for them to be economically viable, whatever the price, even penalisation if necessary.

This way of interpreting community-based care and obliging citizens to take care of each other, with the idea of cutting back on services, is not at all how quartermaking is understood. Quartermakers assume that not everyone is in a position to reciprocate and that reciprocation cannot be a precondition for qualifying as a full citizen. A person's inability to reciprocate cannot be a reason for placing them on the sidelines of society. Quartermaking is used to show hospitality to people who find it difficult to reciprocate. It should be pointed out that this hospitality is unconditional. There is no real need for reciprocity.

Quite a few of the people who are unable to reciprocate actually do have a deep desire to do so, but cannot always find their way to that place. This group certainly contains a large number of 'care avoiders'.

Quite a few people struggle with the fact that there is nothing they can do for others. It feels like they have failed, because they have ended up in a position where all they can do is receive, or take. It feels like they have little or no meaning for others. They have the sense that they are only important to healthcare professionals, or that all they can do is accept other people's charity. The more isolated they get the more bitter they become, because they are unable to generate reciprocity.

Through his understanding of humanity, i.e., that people have a longing to belong, to be reciprocal, the quartermaker aims to realise a different kind of society, in which reciprocity is possible. A quartermaker thinks about changing society's structures and organisations, to make reciprocity more accessible to all. This is because empowering people and strengthening their social position is not enough to induce the desired change. Quartermakers can retain the important idea of reciprocity by finding or creating systems in which non-automatic reciprocity can arise. In the process, quartermakers work towards changing the political system. They look for a society that is organised along different lines, through which reciprocity becomes possible. We might ask ourselves if this kind of systemic change can be achieved in a neoliberal economic system.

An alternative currency has developed in two areas of Ghent in recent years. 'Torekes' (in the district of Rabot) and 'Pluimen' (in the district of Ledeberg). Both are payment systems, subsidised by the city to encourage people to create a nicer, tidier and more liveable neighbourhood. People are paid in the currency if they create a wall garden. They can also earn payments in the currency by working on certain projects designed to give the community a boost (being a reading buddy for children, keeping an elderly lady company, car sharing, keeping a petanque court, helping neighbours cook or do their shopping, coaching a local kids' football team...). The projects are listed in a brochure along with work opportunities and shops and social restaurants where the currency is accepted. The currency can even be used to pay the rent on allotments. It creates a small-scale economy that gives vulnerable people the opportunity to earn a little extra on the side. The system helps improve access to reciprocal relationships. It helps raise people's self-worth, because it gives them a sense of being meaningful to others, of their efforts being appreciated. It results in a better community, and in relationships which are perceived as valuable and important. The fact that these actions are rooted in the community gives them a firmer hold in the immediate environment.

The phenomenon of *bartering* is interesting in that it is also about the improvement of social contact. The system works like this: with *bartering* you become a member of a local group, in which people do things for each other. It's a sort of return to the old system of trading, but in activities rather than goods. The nice thing about these activities is that they often involve others, and each person supports the other in the process. In these local groups, people get to know each other through doing things for each other. The internet facilitates exchanges between existing groups and makes it possible to move beyond the local circle. In this way, ties of friendship can be created through reciprocity. People can offer to do something for others of their own account. Health professionals can strengthen this reciprocity by carrying out tasks with their clients for other citizens. Quartermakers happily use the internet and more particularly social media to find pathways that were formerly much less accessible.

New ideas on finding jobs for people with mental ill health are especially welcome. Work is a meaningful occupation for many people. A person with a good job feels good and enjoys a sense of belonging. Work is often the biggest obstacle for people with mental ill health. The skills are often intact, but maintaining the effort over the long term may be a problem. Our present economic model does not seem well-adapted to people with mental ill health. Indeed, it often seems to cause mental ill health. In the past, a great many training courses, preparatory courses and so on were designed to raise people to a standard that would enable them to cope with a regular job. Some politicians spend a great deal of time developing strategies to encourage people back to work by penalising them financially. Often under the slogan of activation.

In the context of quartermaking (changing the environment, so that people rediscover a place in the new environment), we would like to mention another economy, another business culture, which helps people with mental ill health find their way back to work.

In our present society working and earning money are synonymous with greater prosperity and happiness. A study by the British economist Richard Layard (lecturer at the London School of Economics) (Layard, 2006) showed that since the Second World War people have become 12 times richer, but not happier, and perhaps unhappier. Our society is steeped in the notion of economic return. The question is, what would happen if work and society were based on values other than numerical return and personal benefit. What would happen if solidarity and equality were reinforced, and greed, individualism and disrespect were frowned upon? How would you create well-being and happiness, and what would be the return? This is precisely what Layard's 'happiness economics' set out to show. How do you de-emphasise a company's profits and emphasise its meaning to society, its workers and the local environment? Young people tend to base their choice of career on the social significance of the work. Layard goes into the relationship between economic prosperity and happiness. He believes that we are seeing a worldwide movement towards well-being. This has arisen through disenchantment with the fruits of economic growth and the observation that greater prosperity does not lead to greater happiness.

In his *Handboek betekenisvol ondernemen* (2016) [The Meaningful Entrepreneur's Handbook], business adviser Kees Klomp writes that the purpose economy is the fourth in human history. He is referring here to the work of Aaron Hurst. After the agrarian economy (land possession) came the industrial economy (mass production), followed by the knowledge economy (computer and internet). And now we have arrived at the *purpose economy*.

The purpose economy shifts the emphasis from prosperity to well-being. It involves a better sense of well-being. According to Klomp, the purpose economy is an economy in which business value is determined by what you, the individual or company, mean to society. The more meaningful your company is to society, the more valuable it is. Due to the shift to well-being, we no longer think it important for businesses to generate astronomical profits. If these profits are made at the expense of everyone else, then the company is actually making a loss. A business profit is still useful, but only if it comes through positive social impact.

Aaron Hurst (2014) talks about the switch to a happiness economy. As he sees it, we are on the cusp of a new economy, in which profitability is put to work for human happiness. There are very real doubts over the idea that greater prosperity brings greater happiness. For a long time the maximisation of profit, making as much money as possible, looked like the path the happiness. With happiness as the goal now, instead of money, people are reaching new understandings, even in economic terms. Aaron Hurst saw how people all around him began to attach more importance to sharing (such as car sharing) and making their own products. All of these changes have a common thread: they lead to better relations between people, personal growth and personal experiences. Hurst concluded that we are transitioning to a fourth economy.

In *Rendement van geluk* [Return on Happiness], a report by the *VPRO's Tegenlicht* programme (aired on 3 April 2016), it was said that a new set of business morals emerged at the end of the banking crisis, in which 'social purpose', 'well being' and 'happiness' again play a greater role. Whereas before the standard was *social enterprise*, now *socially responsible enterprise* is the important thing. This means that business should not in any way be harmful. But the future is about *enterprise for social improvement*. This is what businesses do when they generate profit for humanity and the planet and keep a little of the money for themselves at the end of the journey. These are the companies of the future.

The purchase of a product is seen as a political or social transaction. When I buy an organically grown carrot, I make a statement. *Etsy* is a marketplace for people who make things. You buy from craftsperson directly, who makes item with love. By using the product you feel a connection with the maker.

The maker has meaning for the buyer. Buying is a meaningful experience. In the information economy, real contact is lost. Social media gives the illusion of contact but real contact is lost, and social capital diminishes. This is what inspired the movement towards the purpose economy. People want real contact, not Facebook likes or texts. They want things that feel real, they want tight-knit relations. The millennium generation is the first to place meaning at number one. You see more and more CEOs saying that consumption and work patterns are changing radically among the millennium generation. They believe that products and services are not about consumption, but about purpose and valuable experience. They look at work differently, and they look for careers that offer prospects for growth, meaning and real contact. They do not want to be robots. They have come to see that you are the director of your own company. And, just as companies hire and fire, you have to pursue your own wishes and take control of your own career. Freelancers develop their own portfolios and decide who they do or do not want to work for. What they are actually saying is: I won't be bound by a single employer, I will decide what I do for myself. They opt for flexibility.

The *purpose economy* wants to see happiness in the now, while you work. It is about being proud of your life and connected to the people you wish to be associated with. The goal is to strengthen, stimulate and connect people. Purposeful entrepreneurs do not begin with an idea, but a social problem. This is a new paradigm. They start from a problem that they are affected by and want to solve, and then they figure out a business in the process. The primary objective of that business is to solve the problem.

We are talking about ecological and social profit. It is about exceeding your own interests and putting the general interests first. Purpose, giving meaning to what you do, can be about having social contact with others, but also about wanting to learn new things, or to go travelling. The bigger picture is equally important, such as respect for the environment or tackling social injustice. An important starting point, in taking these problems on, is the ability to identify with them at a personal level. This economy places a high value on compassion and sympathy, the ability to immerse yourself in someone else's problem.

Happiness and equity are more important that profit. Customer, producer and staff are a community in which everyone is of equal value.

In this 'purpose economy' the part that emphases the elimination of social inequality is extremely interesting because it ties in with the philosophy behind quartermaking. Companies set themselves up to be accessible by groups of people who would not otherwise find employment.

In the 1980s, Yonkers, New York was rife with criminality, drug addition, prostitution and mugging. One of its residents, Roshi Bernie Glassman, set up a cookie factory: Greyston Bakery (Michael Pirson, 2020). The employees were former drug dealers, rough sleepers and prostitutes from the impoverished surroundings, who were given the opportunity to build a new life. The brownies they make in the Greyston Bakery are used in Ben and Jerry's ice cream. They operate an 'open hiring' system at Greyston. This means no interview for anyone who finds it hard to get a job. No questions asked. The core values are trust and openness.

In their isolation, people with mental ill health often just want to do the sort of things that most people do. By getting away from outsider status they regain social recognition:

> (free translation) The sense of well being increases in many clients when they are functioning in an environment that satisfies the generally acceptable social standards. This sort of environment reflects positively on their persona; to some extent their self-image and self-esteem take the colour of that more highly appreciated environment.
>
> (Van Weeghel in Kal, 2001, p. 52)

Therefore most people with mental ill health just want to belong and to play their part in society. So we could say that a model society that was designed to concentrate on eradicating social inequality would be a society that was accessible to its most vulnerable members.

In this sense, a society which gets its economic support from a purpose society would be a more hospitable society. The existence of a society of this kind would ease the quartermaker's task of enabling the individual to connect. This is why it is important for quartermakers to work towards these structural changes at a higher level. Quartermakers would then be able to work with business leaders in setting up businesses based on the principles of the purpose economy. They would be able to help business leaders gain an understanding of the difficulties experienced by people with mental ill health. The creativity emerging through this collaboration would give rise to companies that provide paid employment for people with mental ill health.

An interesting project that ran as a pilot in Flanders until June 2014, was *Compool*. It developed a pool of skills to put people to work:

> (free translation) In the 'Compool' project (2012–2014) we tried to innovate the employment for people with a chronic disorder. In this project a pool of people with comparable skills was created for a specific job. If an employee decides to leave temporarily for health reasons, someone else is brought in from the pool to continue the job. This gives the employer the guarantee that the work will be done and the employee the guarantee of a temporary break without fear of losing his job.
>
> (Neyens and Van Audenhove, 2015)

165

The project aims to change how the work is organised, thereby opening a path to sustainable employment, and to expand the individual capacities of people with chronic illnesses. The basic principle is to group employees in a pool of competencies; hence the project's name. These employees could easily stand in for each other if one were temporarily unable to work. The interesting thing is that the job coach comes to work at the same place as the person s/he coaches, as this gives her/him a better picture of how that person is performing the job. The project applies the IPS (Individual placement and support) principle. Of greatest significance here is the 'place then train' element: employees are trained in the workplace, on the job. This training method motivates the employee to keep learning. It is important to bear the interests of the employer as well as those of the employee in mind. Under the principles of quartermaking, support is given to both parties: the party providing the opportunity for inclusion and the party seeking inclusion.

4.10 Quartermaking and Interventive Care

> Not only does neglected vulnerability (no support, no help, no way out, or help even countered) tear the person concerned apart, but it spreads easily as social dissatisfaction and produces more victims.
> – Andries Baart, *De zorgval*, 2013, p. 40

Quite a few people refuse help, precisely because of the lack of reciprocity that comes with healthcare. Some people with mental ill health complain that this reciprocity does not exist at all. They feel threatened and anxious at the idea of being dependent on healthcare professionals. I meet many people who do not want to ask for help, precisely because of the long-term embarrassment brought about by a lack of reciprocity. This situation is often created by carers who want to help and want to provide care. People with mental ill health may assume that the healthcare professional could use or misuse their position of power to have them involuntarily detained or force unwanted medication on them. The biggest 'care avoiders' belong to group of people who are in search of that illusive reciprocity, as a means to escape dependence. Interventive care should be designed essentially to re-enable that reciprocity. Some people have had to care for themselves for years, since childhood, in the most difficult of situations, and now they can only perceive the help they are being offered as an element of doubt over their survival abilities. As a healthcare professional you should have a great deal of respect for this attitude. Quartermaking is about trying to find a role that restores for these people some of the reciprocity that has fallen by the wayside. How can I be of meaning to someone else? A question that we all ask ourselves.

(free translation) Regular attendance at the place where patients stay – also known as presence – is one of the best ways to gain their trust. You gain confidence mostly through action, not through words. When you are present patients can make an informed judgement about what kind of person you are – you don't want to know what patients think of psychiatric practitioners! And by rolling up your sleeves at that point you build trust. It also makes you approachable to the people closest to him and you can gain the trust of that important group of people. 'Be there or be square!'.

(Tielens and Verster, 2010)

This is the basis, but of equal importance is the place where you agree to meet and the point at which you choose to do so in a person's treatment. Below, I give a picture of the coaching provided by a FACT Team, which was given at four different places, based on the stage of the coaching. A trend is observable in the relationship with the healthcare professional, and it is reflected in the meeting places that were agreed. The place at which quartermaking was practised for this client was a vital factor in all further contact.

Florian is on the locked ward of a psychiatric unit, where he is acting in a menacing way and causing concern. The situation becomes so difficult that the practitioner gives him the choice between sedation or discharge. He chooses discharge but is livid at having had the choice forced upon him in this way. He was seeking help, but wanted it on his own terms. The stay on the locked ward had forced him to relinquish control. He seemed to seek help by demanding it. A conflict had arisen over power and control of the healthcare situation. Florian demands that we make more time for him. He is so insistent about this, that we see the situation as threatening. We take it as a signal that he is not in a good place. My colleague in the FACT Team gets a full verbal broadside. Florian threatens her. She feels unsafe and arranges to meet in one of our rooms. She asks a colleague to stay available in an adjacent room. Florian seems to have cottoned on to this. He is on our territory, and he feels in danger. There are several colleagues in the office for safety reasons. This is where he perceives the threat to be. It is as though we have increased the odds, in order to restrain him.

I call Florian. He would like to meet, but it will have to be in a cafeteria in the town centre. Not at his place, not at ours. The conversation in the cafeteria has its ups and downs. He looks like becoming verbally aggressive at times. He says he'll punch me in the gut if he meets me on the street, and that I should be grateful it's him, because, unlike the others, he delivers a clean punch. He talks about healthcare professionals and how they always set conditions when he wants something. They don't listen to him. They don't help him. He is homeless and staying at a friend's for now. He can have another month there, so there is no problem. I listen. I tell him that I don't think a healthcare practitioner should just sit and listen behind a desk. I like to get out and about with people, literally, to find the solutions to problems. I want to be available and to experience my client's problems for myself.

He is glad that breakfast is so cheap here, but when I offer to pay he gets angry again. He buys my breakfast, not the other way round. I have no choice. Obviously, he wants to stay in control of the situation. Letting me get breakfast is a form of surrender. He refuses to be the taker. He will decide when and how often we talk. He has demanded twice a week from my colleague. On leaving I shake his hand. I can't help looking over my shoulder as I return to the office. I am afraid that he will follow me.

Florian has chosen to meet in public. You are among other people, where you observe all the social conventions: a drink together, one of you picks up the bill... The people chatting in a tearoom are bound to abide by the conventions and etiquette of the place. A type of equality prevails, as everyone is on neutral territory.

The situation that he and I found ourselves in, a fraught meeting in public, crops up in films of the kind directed by Alfred Hitchcock. It is how Slavoj Zizek (1992) describes a social dance in the film *Saboteur* (Hitchcock, 1942). In the middle of the festivities we follow two parties: the main character, who is helping his girlfriend escape, and the Nazis. All are at the dance. Both parties rely on not being discovered by the other. This is what they have in common. The parties must keep all of their actions in line with the etiquette of the social dance. They cannot afford to be conspicuous. When one of the Nazis attempts to lead the woman away from the party, the main character, her boyfriend, asks her to dance. The Nazis can do nothing without breaking the rules of the party, and so they are forced to back off. Afterwards they are unable to arrest the host, because he joins a couple and leaves the party with them...

Neither of the parties, who are opponents, can do anything while they are all in a crowd or a group, precisely because they have to follow etiquette. To maintain the stand-off, or the safety of the situation, it is important that the others sitting around are unaware of the tensions between the main characters.

Florian has been involuntarily detained before, and he no longer trusts the health professionals. A meeting in a café puts him at ease. He knows the health professionals will follow a certain etiquette, and that it wouldn't be possible to involuntarily detain a person in the tea room without seriously disturbing the peace. The meeting place gives him control of the situation and offers him safety. Unlike the situation in the film, he is not trying to escape us. He wants to control the situation, so that he can safely decide whether or not we can be trusted. It gives him the time to assess us. Time which is important to us too, in which to meet and make a connection. The healthcare professional shares this feeling of safety when a client sees the need to adhere to social convention. Contact becomes possible thanks to the unwitting third parties, the people sitting around us. This public space is a non-authoritarian field, in which people meet. We pretend that we are having a cosy chat, through which it becomes possible for us to have a cosy chat. It more or less works. Moments of friendliness alternate with moments of verbal aggression. He appears to want to assess me, without making himself too dependent on me. Here, in this situation, at this point of our togetherness, it is important that an ignorant party, the other people seated at tables around us, be present. In the office, where the previous meeting took place, the only other people were colleagues, and they were anything but ignorant, third parties, and this was why he felt threatened.

Three days later, Florian and I meet at the local services centre. We had agreed this place at the end of our last meeting in the tea-room. Florian would like to do voluntary work. He would like to work with elderly people. I feel that I should along with his desire, and that I should come good on my promise to go out and about with him despite his threats at our previous meeting. A few min-utes before our appointment he texts to say that he is waiting at the entrance. We talk. For the first time he talks about his parents, their divorce, his mother's suicide.

We go in and meet a person who describes the volunteer jobs available at the services centre. During this encounter I am sur-prised by my client's social skills. He says there are several jobs he would like to do, but that he also hopes to implement a few of his own ideas. He would like to bring old and young together through folk games. They remind him of his grandmother, whom he loves dearly. He would like to play these games with the elderly who come in throughout the day. Our assistant thinks that this is an excellent idea. The services centre occasionally works with youngsters from the community. Florian, who was so aggressive before, is now a wonderful advocate of connection and conciliation. The services centre assistant says that we can quite happily get to know the elderly folk at the centre. She gives us the heads up about one of them. A difficult man, apparently. It doesn't take us long to real-ise who she is talking about. Our rather careless use of the word 'three cushion' fires him up: 'Who do you think you are? You want to play three-cushion, when for years we've played a different game. Have you any idea what you are saying, or how rude you are? Why don't you have the decency to ask what we play, and then fit in with that?' I laugh, and say that he has a point. I watch for Florian's response, afraid that his aggression might be triggered by this sort of attitude. But Florian is on my wavelength, and not at all defensive. He says that's not how we meant it, and that we are very happy to play billiards by their rules. Later Florian will explain to me that the old guys in the services centre may have felt threatened by what they saw as a couple of young greenhorns coming in and trying to change things. I agree with his assessment and tell him that it's a shrewd insight, and that he knows a lot about people. It brings a marked improvement in our contact.

The grumpy old guy tells us that only one of us can play, not both at the same time. Florian would rather that I play. He wants to watch. I allow the assertive old man to give me a lesson on the game of billiards. He starts joking with me and the others. I go and stand next to Florian occasionally. He nods and smiles.

I call him two days later. He tells me that he returned to the services centre the day after our visit. He adds that it was good to be there together the first time: 'It was important to break the ice.'

Florian and I have created a bond. I promise to call him next week for a new appointment. He tells me that he is starting to worry about not having a home. He is looking for accommodation. I tell him that I will help him find a place. He says that he is running low on friends. He says that people have said they are afraid of him. I am pleased with this opening, and I tell him that I didn't feel all that comfortable when we met in the cafeteria. We talk. We have a bond...

And, in the end, while Florian stays with a girlfriend for a while, and later, when he gets a place of his own, we arrange to meet at his home. He invites me over and I feel entirely safe. Our conversations go well. He reflects on himself and his frequently aggressive way with others, which tends to scare them off.

The places where you meet can be extremely important in establishing a bond of trust with a client, especially if your client is care avoidant. He or she may play the game of wait and see. He/she does not trust you, but is prepared to give you a chance. In the early stages of getting to know you he/she does not dare hope that you will turn out to be reliable, through fear of being soon disappointed again. As a healthcare professional you sometimes have to demonstrate reliability long enough for the care avoider to build up the courage to cross the bridge. You are put to the test. Accompanying the care avoider to places that are important to him/her can bring you closer to achieving your goal. When you are quartermaking (in Florian's case it was about finding somewhere for him to do voluntary work), accompanying the client to these places is a way of establishing a bond with them. It is a way of giving them no reason to be defensive. In this sense quartermaking, recovery and interventive care are one and the same. One does not follow on from another. It is often a combination, a necessary combination.

The home support worker tells me that she can no longer get in touch with Maria. The caretaker at the apartment building says that my client has lost the key to the main entrance, and that she climbs in over the balustrade. The neighbours find it disconcerting. The electricity has been cut off and she eats on the landing, in the glow of the street lights. The neighbours find this disconcerting too. Maria can no longer stay in her home as she hears voices and they threaten her. The next weekend she is picked up by the police as she walks along a busy highway. I coach her on the FACT Team.

She is involuntarily admitted. On my first visit she says that she does not want to see me. She says that she doesn't need anyone to coach her at home. And anyway, her voices have mentioned me by name, and she thinks that I am in danger. For my own safety it is best that I stay away. She says that I should be more concerned with my own family. She talks very briefly about the music she has written, and about the message she is trying to get across in it. It is a very brief conversation. I visit her every two weeks. She refuses all treatment on the ward to which she has been involuntarily admitted. She is administered medication forcibly. After several visits, each a little longer than the last, something in her attitude towards me begins to change. She tells me that she would like to be a peer supporter, and that it is something she would really enjoy. She knows that the work is voluntary. She realises that she needs money, and she would like to look for a paid job. I see opportunities to help her with this and put her in touch with the peer supporter on our team. We have a brilliant conversation, in which Maria talks about her difficulties with the medication forced upon her. The peer supporter has clearly created a bond with her. I get the feeling that everything is on the right track. I get her an appointment with the employment adviser attached to our team. The adviser gives her information on the various pathways for people with disabilities. But Maria would like to find a job through the normal channels. She does not view herself as sick or disabled. She says that she would like to give it a go this way first, and that if it doesn't work she can always try the other ways. We have a fragile connection and to us this is really important. A bond is gradually developing, and we can build on it.

The home support worker, CPAS social services and myself (the home coaches) request a meeting with the team at the psychiatric ward where Maria is staying. The team has greeted her ideas about work and being a peer supporter with distrust. They want her to begin by sticking with the medication, and to realise that she is dealing with psychosis. Maria herself sees more benefit in the contacts established through us, the home support workers, because they address her desire to take her place in society. We, the home support workers, are happy to have found an opening through which we can get to work with her.

At a new meeting the ward team appear to go all out for a confrontation with Maria. They are of the opinion that she will only get better by taking her medication and spending more time on the ward. The team spokesman says that it is still too early for other things like job seeking. The consultation ends in a standoff. A few days later I get an angry phone call from someone on Maria's ward team. Maria has been prevented from contacting peer supporters, including the peer supporter on our team. If she becomes a peer supporter they fear that she will advise patients to stop taking their medication.

I plead with them again to cooperate in some way, by allowing the various members of the network to adopt different positions and take different viewpoints. The difference can actually give rise to a wonderful dynamic, which may ultimately lead to a compromise that is acceptable to all, especially Maria. However, the ward team is clearly a very hierarchical structure. They are not used to accommodating different opinions. I get a call from the lady from social services, who was there for the consultation with Maria. She tells me that the psychiatrist, who was not present at the team meeting, but obviously holds the reins, is very cross with me.

A few days later I call the psychiatrist myself, in the hope of talking things through. She says that she is not cross with me, but furious. When I say that in that case we should talk it over, she replies that she does not wish to invest her time in that sort of conversation. In her opinion there is nothing to discuss. Further discussion is a waste of time.

I hear later, from my manager, that the psychiatrist had complained to her director about me, and that he in turn had contacted the centre where I work. Fortunately, my managers have every confidence in me and support my views on recovery and quartermaking. These vertically aligned and hierarchically organised structures can assert themselves powerfully when you stand up for your clients' interests.

I tell Maria that I will keep in touch with her when her detention comes to an end. She gives it a little thought and smiles. There is something else that she would like me to do for her: find a reliable psychic. She wants to stay in touch with me about this.

We agree to meet at her home. She prefers to go to the park across the road. She lies down in the grass. The ground feels a little too cold for me so I sit on a bench. She doesn't answer my questions. I say nothing. After half an hour of silence, lying on her back and gazing up at the tree, she says that it is lovely in the park. I say that trees can be incredibly beautiful. She agrees, and tells me she wants a man. The psychic. She wants him to be a man. Then a long talk begins, in which tells me all about her psychotic experiences.

And so a connection can be established with Maria, another 'care avoider', by looking into a few practicalities, such as peer support training and a paid job. I aim to put her in touch with other people who can collaborate on the answers to these questions. Through quartermaking, you can set up social contact and persons of trust. As a healthcare professional you enter a partnership with the client, and that partnership can open a route to discussing other difficulties. Obviously, healthcare professionals who do not personally see the value of this method can seriously obscure the route to quartermaking and recovery, or even block it altogether. Especially if they occupy a position of power.

Quartermaking and inspiring compassion in the client's immediate environment are important when clients themselves appear capable of talking about their suffering. If they are unable to talk about themselves they become even more vulnerable to exclusion. The 'inexpressible suffering' and 'indescribable discord' that go with it – terms used by Jean-Francois Lyotard (Jacob Michael Held, 2005) – can leave the other party entirely unaware of the problem, so that attention must be drawn to it by an intermediary, someone who speaks on behalf of the person who is unable to express their own suffering. It is only logical for people who stare into space after exchanging a few brief sentences to be avoided. So too are people who keep asking the same question without listening to the answer. In these cases, it seems that normal contact is impossible; people do not have the means by which to describe their own suffering. There is no metalanguage to discuss their relationship or lack of relationship with others. There are no words to describe the solitude that results from a lack of communication. Anyone who spends time with these people and discovers the person behind the 'difficult contact', will notice that they have a need for contact too. You can tell this from a smile. You can sense it from the sudden question: 'When are you coming back?' You can feel it in the handshake when you leave, and in the softly spoken 'thank you'. The solitude that comes from people's suffering increases that very suffering... The work of the quartermaker is (free translation) 'to make the speechless heard' (Kal, 2001, p. 60).

> (free translation) That brings us to something of an impasse. Can space be made for an indescribable difference? In other words: can you offer space to someone you cannot 'place'? The link between the speechless and public is sought here in the concept of hospitality.
>
> (Kal, Ibid., p. 60)

The quartermaker succeeds in being there for the client by experiencing their exclusion with them. You become a bit of a nomad yourself, a person without territory. The quartermaker can occupy or sense the position of isolation without succumbing to the anxiety and uncertainty that it brings. S/he can share the negative experiences, but can also experience the positives. S/he thinks that the uniqueness of the position, not being one of the masses, should be cherished. The quartermaker is also able to be amazed by this disposition, without romanticising or idealising it. A quartermaker is capable of sharing a feel for all its subtleties. And with this feel s/he too can be something of an outsider, but with a good, firm stance that allows him or her to keep in touch with the environment for the client. It is important that the quartermaker represent the patient's interests, but in a way that ensures s/he does not isolate him/herself from others in the patient's environment. S/he should not be so defensive or confrontational in defence of the patient's interests that the environment shrinks away and the quartermaker isolates himself/herself or undermines his or her position with others. It is often a delicate balance. A quartermaker who identifies solely with the place of the outsider, often hospitals, and is therefore unable to establish a connection with others in the patient's environment will bind the patient to him/her and the organisation, and this can lead to a prolonged stay in hospital and to chronification.

A quartermaker is also capable of grasping chance opportunities. You develop a long attention span in your work, which makes you ever ready to take advantage of good situations as and when they occur. This means that your work is guided by a theme, that you remember the history of your work with the client, can accommodate the present and theorise about the future.

A quartermaker always has this feeling of hospitality in his/her attitude, wherever s/he goes, irrespective of any particular patient. This gives him/her the ability to meet people who are very unlike him/her. It creates opportunities for new encounters, especially with people outside the mental healthcare setting. Through these new meetings s/he increases the chances of potential connections which s/he can later use to the benefit of the people s/he coaches. He or she expands their own network for the benefit of present and future clients. A love of animals can play an important role in this.

Due to the voices in her head, her dog was the only being in whom Ella could take comfort, the only being that gave or received something akin to human love. On her last admission, which she had put off as long as she possibly could, she had to take the little dog to the pound. It was an awful, heart-rending moment. In our conversations Ella speaks of the animal with great fondness. Is it still alive? She misses it terribly, but hopes that it is doing well, that it has gone to a good home. Our first objective on this admission is to find out what has become of her dog.

The lady at the pound knows that the dog was homed, but is unable to tell us where. It is against the rules. But she is deeply affected by our story and is prepared to do something special for us: she will ask the lady who now owns the dog to get in touch with us.

The new owner lives about thirty kilometres from the hospital. Ella and I go together in the car. It's a wonderful reunion. The dog recognises her immediately and happily jumps up on her. The new owner is an elderly lady who lives alone and looks after the dog very well. She is a little lonely herself and very happy to have us visit. She has coffee ready, and has bought a cake. Ella talks about the dog's habits, its likes and dislikes. The new owner agrees instantly. I have never seen Ella speak to anyone else this much. The new owner is very pleased with the information and will keep it in mind.

I take Ella to visit the woman a few more times. We always take the dog for a little walk. On these walks Ella and I establish a relationship of trust, and this makes it possible for her to talk about her psychotic episodes. I often think back to those afternoons with Ella and the dog's new owner, with coffee and cake, and to the dog, which Ella always described as 'my little dog'.

A quartermaker is a good negotiator. He or she can use their own energies and abilities as a bargaining chip in creating opportunities for patients to connect. If a potential landlord wavers about a client, the quartermaker can put him/herself or another party forward as a home supporter for the would-be tenant, thereby allowing the landlord to discriminate positively when awarding the tenancy agreement.

In Belgium, quartermakers draw political attention to systemic discrimination against people with mental ill health and are in a position to work with politicians to eliminate this discrimination. Several colleagues and I visit the MP Valerie Van Peel (N-VA [New Flemish Alliance]). We criticise her proposal to force people to seek help for their addictions by removing their benefits. We also point out that many of those who seek an admission and actually want to do something about their problems are being refused by services because the issue is too complex and difficult.

Quartermakers can do some fine work through social media. I have a Facebook page on which I regularly report on my quartermaking and recovery work. It puts me in touch with peer supporters and professionals in Belgium and the Netherlands, and it is also a way of contacting volunteers to work on our ward. I am aware that while Facebook is a powerful medium for reaching out and connecting with people, it can also be misused to exclude people with mental ill health.

> She stands a little vacantly in her dressing gown, in the middle of the station concourse. I can't really tell the expression on her face. The camera is too far away. She has noticed the photographer, that much is certain. They must have had very brief contact. The photograph is on a Facebook page, a 'fan page', or so its creators call it, entitled: 'Station Lady', and it is preceded by the name of the city in question. She is homeless. The anonymous creators of this Facebook page want her to stay on living at the station. She has already been deported once as she is not of Belgian nationality.
>
> The profile photo is a stylised drawing, which depicts her crouching. Behind her, a stylised poop. This is in reference to a genuine article in the regional section of one of the newspapers. They report that the woman is causing a nuisance. The article is illustrated by a photograph, which shows her crouching over the gutter to do her business.
>
> The dressing gown photograph was submitted in response to a call for 'zwerfies' or humiliating photos. The more compromising a position the person is caught in, the more points the page's creators award the photographer.
>
> This photo carries the caption: 'Haters gonna hate'. This is slang for the idea that whatever you do you will be criticised, so you might as well do what you want. The page's creators think it is funny, apparently, to make this woman a figure of provocation, as provocative, perhaps, as their infringement of good taste. Only it is at her expense. On a separate events page, announcing a genuine fan day at the station, a good 1100 people have indicated (probably in jest) their intention to come along and party with the woman. A few animations, inspired by her photographs, turn her into a break-dancer or the victim of police arrest. A competition is announced to discover her name. Someone replies that his uncle met her in a shelter once, and that she is actually schizophrenic.
>
> The page's creators develop a webshop with all kinds of merchandise, such as buttons and T-shirts showing the stylised image of the woman and a reference to the Facebook page. The kitchen apron reads: 'We eat from the bins here.' An awful lot of youngsters see the hilarity of it all and like the page. In fact, it has more than

1200 likes. Some, judging by their responses, have realised that the page goes beyond the bounds of decency. But all add some witticism or other to show their sympathy for the provocation. Someone makes a reference to Brussels, "where more of the stinkers live". I see just two comments criticising the page's creators.

Once I have seen the page I can't erase the words or the pictures from my mind. Who would do something like that? Who is behind it? Why are so many youngsters amused by what I, my colleagues and friends, find so horrifying? And, moreover, will I be able to show those youngsters that their actions are least pleasant of all to the homeless lady? As a quartermaker, I try to create space in society for people with mental ill health. This is almost antiquartermaking: creating a fellowship, a community, to isolate and exclude a person on the basis of their difference.

As a quartermaker you are always trying to get through to people who exclude others on the basis of their difference. But you don't want to make the mistake of excluding them through your response. Two of my colleagues and I contact the creators through the chat function on the Facebook page. We agree to meet in the city. But they don't show up. I continue to ask them, through my own page, to get in touch with us. They decline to respond to any of our communication. In the meantime, I report the page to Facebook, but to no avail. Facebook tells me that the page is not in breach of their bullying or privacy rules. I contact the city council and the privacy commission. There is nothing that they can do either. At a meeting of the Flemish Working Group on Quartermaking we decide to all respond to the Facebook page at once (about eighty of us). We also send the page's creators an invitation to talk to us. We call on them to employ their creativity for the benefit of homeless people. In the end, Facebook bows to the pressure and takes the page down.

At no point do the page's creators ever relinquish their anonymity. A real discussion is never had, which I think is a pity. I think too of all those youngsters, who couldn't see that the page went far beyond the bounds of decency and was nothing more, nothing less, than a serious invasion of a person's privacy, a person who hadn't chosen to be in the public eye.

It is a shame that we were unable to talk to them about the page. It turned the homeless woman into a sort of cartoon figure. In other words, the stylisation and dehumanisation of her photograph lengthened the distance of the relationship. That distance from the homeless woman made it easier to see the mockery as painless.

Homelessness does not give others the right to abuse the public nature of a private life that a person has not chosen for themselves. To be homeless is to be doomed, through circumstance, to a life in public, without privacy. In this sense, we need solutions for homelessness. Our next step was to set up consultations with a variety of authorities, such as the police and city services, the NMBS national railway staff and healthcare professionals. We agreed on a plan to ensure that this woman would not simply be left to her fate. Homelessness calls for solutions, and, if solutions can be found, there is a chance that people will stop supporting these stigmatising Facebook pages.

7th May 2013. Participants start queuing early for the quartermaking workshop in Ghent. We, the organisers (professionals, local residents and peer supporters), have been planning this day for a year. There are between 350 and 400 participants. It is an unexpected success. A highly diverse audience of students, (former) psychiatric patients, peer supporters, local residents, politicians, professionals, police representatives ... descends from every province in Flanders. Ghent presents itself on that day as a very open and social city that offers a great many initiatives for those who live on the edge of society. I am fortunate to be given the opportunity to interview Doortje Kal, after which we are surrounded by peer supporters, who speak about their quartermaking experiences. Many of the speakers refer to her book as a benchmark for their work. The comments afterwards are full of praise. They describe an encouraging meeting, a warm atmosphere, full of hope and prospects for integration. I look back with satisfaction on a pleasing day, on which some of the toughest and most beautiful experiences in my many years of quartermaking were crystallised. The meetings with Doortje Kal were the high points. She gave me a language with which to explain what I do, a language that makes me more specific and effective in my quartermaking work.

The workshop led to the foundation of the Ghent Working Group on Quartermaking, which was attended by healthcare professionals in and outside the psychiatric system, as well as psychiatric patients and their families, people with mental ill health in general, and services concerned with poverty, job centres, home support workers, and people from halfway houses, cultural centres, local politicians and local residents. This work is picked up by people from the Flemish Association for Mental Health, and in 2015 the Flemish Working Group on Quartermaking is set up as part of the recovery platform. I chair the meetings. The local organiser invites local healthcare professionals, patients, patient relatives, peer supporters and local residents. Wherever possible we try to meet at locations outside the mental healthcare setting. We encourage people to look beyond their compartments and to seek out collaborations. It is often about getting to know new organisations and ideas to promote quartermaking, but also a laboratory for creating new ways to enable people with mental ill health to reconnect. The meetings also inspire social action, as did the meeting in Ostend, where we managed through collective action to have an extremely discriminatory Facebook group taken off the internet. In fact, at that meeting it is stated clearly for the first time that all attendees will view themselves in the first place as citizens, and that the healthcare professionals among them will ask themselves, as citizens, how hospitable their own clubs and associations are to the people they care for through the day.

Doortje Kal attends these meetings regularly. She enjoys being with us and feels every meeting the friendliness of the people in the meeting We hope that we will get to see more and more quartermakers at work, and that they will continue to focus on the individual and political level, as well as the societal level.

We assume that, as the number of psychiatric beds decreases, the hospitality extended to people with mental ill health will become an even more important aspect of care and that the thinking on quartermaking will be even more strongly tied to the thinking on how society in general should be organised.

Roel De Cuyper (ex-director of the Psychiatric Centre) gives pride of place to quartermaking at the Ghent workshop:

> Quartermaking (...) can lead to a conscious citizenship, which can be interwoven with care for the other, for Levinas's 'small goodness'. This may even lead to a slight collective resistance, needed more than ever today. I would like to encourage you all to civil disobedience against a society built along neoliberal lines, not through misplaced defiance, but, among other things, by placing quartermaking on the agenda for a broad social debate.

References

Andries Baart and Christa Carbo, *De zorgval. Analyse, kritiek en uitzicht*, Amsterdam, Thoeris, 2013.

Jos Ten Berge, Beyond outsiderism. In *Marginalia. Perspectives on outsider art*, Zwolle (ed.), De Stadshof Museum Foundation, pp. 78–90, 2000.

James Brett, *De Standaard*, 3 March 2016.

Gail Brown, Building community through self-awareness and self-expression. In Luisa Del Giudice (ed.), *Sabato Rodia's towers in watts. Arts, migrations, development*, New York, Fordham University Press, pp. 327–336, 2015.

Roger Cardinal, *Outsider art*, Westport Connecticut, Praeger, 1972.

Jacques Derrida, *Over gastvrijheid*, Amsterdam, Boom, 1998.

Steve Dow, *James Brett and the museum of everything*, Collingwood, Art Guide Australia, 2017.

R.E. Drake, D.R. Becker, R.E. Clark, K.T. Mueser, Research on the individual placement and support model of supported employment. *Psychiatric Quarterly*, 70, 289–301, 1999.

Jeff Feuerzeig and Henry S. Rosenthal, *The devil and Daniel Johnston* documentary, 2005.

John Foot, *The man who closed the asylums, Franco Basaglia and the revolution in Mental Health Care*, London and New York, VersoBooks, 2015.

Jonathan Franzen, Imperial bedroom. *The New Yorker*, October 5, 1998.

Ervin Goffman, *Stigma: Notes on the management of spoiled identity*, London, Penguin, 1990 (1963).

Jacob Michael Held, Expressing the inexpressible, Lyotard and the differend. *Journal of the British Society for Phenomenology*, 36(1), 76–89, 2005.

Hannah Höch, Diary entry, 11 September 1937. First published in Ralf Burmeister and Eckhard Fürlus (eds.), *Hannah Höch – Eine Lebenscollage*, vol. II/2, Ostfildern-Ruit, 1995.

Aaron Hurst, *The purpose economy, How your desire for impact, personal growth and community is changing the world*, Boise Idaho, Elevate, 2014.

Luce Irigaray, *Ik, jij, wij. Voor een cultuur van het onderscheid*, Kampen, Kok Agora, 1992.

Doortje Kal, *Kwartiermaken. Werken aan ruimte voor mensen met een psychiatrische achtergrond*, Amsterdam, Boom, 2001.

Doortje Kal, Rutger Post and Gerda Scholtens, *Meedoen gaat niet vanzelf. Kwartiermaken in theorie en praktijk*, Amsterdam, Tobi Vroegh, 2012.

Doortje Kal, *Verder met Kwartiermaken. Naar de verwelkoming van het verschil*, Amsterdam, Tobi Vroegh, 2013.

Richard Layard, *Happiness: Lessons from a new science*, London, Penguin Books, 2006.

red. Heinz Mölders, W. van de Graaf, M. Janssen, *Versterkende gesprekken*, Amsterdam, Uitgeverij Tobi Vroegh, 2017, pp. 81–102.

Inge Neyens and Chantale Van Audenhove, Compool. Een zoektocht naar een innovatieve arbeidsorganisatie voor mensen met een chronische aandoening. In *Over.Werk. Tijdschrift van het Steunpunt WSE*, Leuven, Work and Social Economy Resource Centre, Den Haag, Acco, 2015–2025, pp. 14–21.

Marius Nuy, *De nacht van Nederland*, Amsterdam, SWP, 2001.

Michael Pirson, Restoring dignity with open hiring, Greyston Bakery and the recognition of value. *Rutgers Business Review*, 5(2), 236–247, 2020.

M. Rutenfrans-Stupar, M.T. Van Regenmortel and R. Schalk, How to enhance social participation and well-being in (formerly) homeless clients: A structural equation modelling approach. *Social Indicators Research*, 145, 329–348, 2019. https://doi.org/10.1007/s11205-019-02099-8.

Selma Sevenhuijsen, De plaats van zorg. Over de relevantie van zor-gethiek voor sociaal beleid, lecture at the University of Utrecht, 2000, quoted in Doortje Kal 'Meedoen gaat niet vanzelf', p. 63.

Jules Tielens and Maurits Verster, *Bemoeizorg*, Utrecht, De Tijdstroom, 2010.

Ans van Berkum, *Willem van Genk, A marked man and his world*, Zwolle, Waanders Drukkers, 1998.

Rudi Visker, *Vreemd gaan en vreemd blijven. Filosofie van de multiculturaliteit*, Amsterdam, Boom, 2005.

C. Wang and M.A. Burris, Photovoice: Concept, methodology, and use for participatory needs assessment. *Health Education and Behaviour*, 24(3), 369–387, 1997.

Slavoj Zizek, *Looking Awry: An introduction to Jacques Lacan through popular culture*, Cambridge MA, October Books, 1992.

5

CONCLUSION
Psychiatry in Recovery

Today, the places where people were supported for many years have disappeared. Rooms, therapy areas, chapels... gone for good. And yet, where the sky now shows through the gap, we can still imagine the original walls. We even see the interior. We see ourselves walking through the corridors, opening doors and closing them again behind us. It is a vague picture, and we cannot quite make out the details. But we can still feel what it was like to walk through them.

My colleague Hilde watches the demolition of our old institution with some patients and local residents. The building was not up to the current safety standards. As the demolition progresses, Hilde spots an opportunity for remembrance and has a word with the crane operator. She points to the stained glass window. The man does not understand much English. He makes a sign to say that he will do his best. Bystanders watch in mild excitement and anticipation. Hilde takes a photo. The grappling arms work slowly and carefully, conscious of their power, bringing an overall feeling of tenderness to the operation. A few bricks fall to the ground before the window comes free of the partly demolished wall. The crane driver hands the gem proudly to Hilde. She puts it somewhere safe, awaiting its new role. A little of the old will be preserved in the new. Something precious from the past will live on in this window.

I see the stained glass window as a symbol of the healthcare professional's presence, and of the quartermaker's work, I see it as a symbol of the healthcare worker who makes it his or her job to establish connections and, above all, as a symbol of the care provider as the provider of hope. Healthcare professionals who are present also help the people in their care to counter an admission's harmful side effects, the walls, the obstacles in the way of recovery. The stained glass window is the chink in the wall, where the light enters from outside.

Interactions that aid recovery will have to be teased from a psychiatric system that rests on the depersonalisation of people through diagnosis. Can the walls be demolished to free the stained glass windows? Can psychiatry take a new path, in keeping with its new societal role?

DOI: 10.4324/9781003220015-6

Can psychiatry recover too? Can it occupy a meaningful new place in the changing social attitudes to mental ill health? And if so, how? Can it evolve towards greater societal participation and place its own importance in context by transferring some of its tasks to people outside its walls? This will certainly be a challenge, especially when innovations such as more care in the community take hold. There is no way back. The reduction in beds is already under way. Some people in the psychiatric system cling to how it used to be. The history of psychiatry is one of isolation and exclusion. Ideas still circulate in which 'isolation' and 'confinement' are seen as restorative, and they are often clothed in wonderful-sounding, philosophical and poetic phrases and linked to ideologies that fail to acknowledge the opinion of the patient. Practitioners hold onto the past and resist. They are in denial about what went wrong, what still goes wrong and what has been done to people. Criticism from patients and former patients is still often met with resistance. In the worst cases, their criticisms are even ascribed to their illness. This utterly disqualifies them as partners in the discussion. People do not want the old buildings to be demolished. The stained glass window, the future remembrance of something beautiful and valuable, is still fixed in the old, bare walls they are so desperate to preserve.

The question is one of how psychiatry, as a system, survives this process of change. A vast expertise was amassed in the psychiatric institution, and it can be put to good use in offering treatment outside the institution, in the home. The psychiatric system can decentralise by putting its help and support at the disposal of healthcare professionals and clients outside the institution. The important thing here is to separate the bed, the coaching and the treatment. Beds on prescription are still in short supply. These beds are offered without treatment. Clients are given a bed in a psychiatric unit for a short period of time, with no intake procedure and the minimum of red tape. The importance of the telephone on prescription was soon recognised on our ward. After leaving the ward a person can still phone in, and one of the nurses will take the time to listen. People sometimes call when they come under additional stress, but at other times it is just to share some good news.

The psychiatric system could also offer all kinds of group services, independent of the admissions. This could be a substantial addition to day centres, which at present are geared mostly towards leisure time activities. But it could just as easily involve family counselling. It may also be important to take care of the simple things, like making the cafeteria more inviting for local residents. Once, we had the idea of setting up a laundry service on the grounds of the institution, so that local residents would be more inclined to pop in. Ideas like these would help open and improve access to psychiatry, and that in itself would have a destigmatising effect.

Psychiatry's recovery lies in doing things on a smaller scale. Small units of healthcare professionals who no longer lodge in the institutions, but live in the neighbourhood itself, as well as professionals who visit people in their homes. Day centres, halfway houses and recovery academies are widespread, and they are independent of the psychiatric institution. As long as safety cannot be guaranteed for people with mental ill health, we will need places where people with similar experiences can meet and support each other. There is a real need for care hotels, run by people with experience, to offer people a brief relaxing stay, a breather, or perhaps even prevent admission to a psychiatric institution.

But more importantly, it seems to me, psychiatry can recover by accepting and internalising a new attitude. Mental healthcare can broaden its base in the community by exercising a little humility in its dealings with organisations that have already done much in this area. By suddenly trying to find a niche in society, from which to treat people with mental health problems, psychiatry is hardly doing anything new. By reducing its size, literally and figuratively, it can do good work precisely by cooperating with other organisations. As and when the reduction in beds increases the pressures in other areas, such as night shelters in the cities, the expertise in psychiatry can be used to offer support in these areas too. That expertise will also prove vital in the provision of more, affordable rental accommodation and the organisation of smaller-scale projects, in cooperation with social housing agencies, as a way of offering support to the new tenants, the new citizens, those who vacated the psychiatric system along with the healthcare providers, as well as landlords and other tenants. This is as helpful to the clients as it is to the societal organisations that concern themselves with these clients. The mental healthcare system has a caring and supportive presence, along with the organisations that handle these tasks.

It is important for the psychiatric institute to give more responsibility to its employees. Allowing healthcare professionals to work in different organisations should help towards 'decompartmentalisation'. Collaborations between organisations are more efficient when there is an exchange of personnel. Given more mobility and experience of different workplaces, healthcare professionals will be less inclined to compartmentalise. A trainee placement on a FACT Team or a similar group in other geographical locations would be beneficial for every psychiatric healthcare professional. It would help them recognise the tunnel vision that sets in for a healthcare practitioner in a psychiatric institution. A tunnel vision that often underestimates the strength of patient self-management, precisely because of the perspective you get in a place where self-management is taken away.

People in the new mental healthcare system in the Netherlands speak about the importance of digitisation, and not just the forums and websites for peer communication and consultation. Digitisation can also aid the development of systems through which the client can manage his or her own records or new communities of people can be formed. Because of this, it presents a solution to the concerns about privacy. The client has control.

Can the mental healthcare professional be in a recovery process? A healthcare professional's recovery involves letting go of his or her traditional education, which stresses diagnoses and professional distance. Letting go of the ward rules as the main framework of reference causes uncertainty and concern for some healthcare professionals. Some will interpret the new emphasis as a loss. Gradually, however, they will learn to fill their roles in a different way. The healthcare professional will learn that self-management is important for the patient. I know that quite a few healthcare professionals feel liberated by this new approach, for it allows them to reveal more of themselves through their patient contact.

Obviously, our education should reflect these changes. I remember a time when supervisors greeted interns with a degree of suspicion for choosing to work in psychiatry. They would be asked some very probing questions about their past, because it was assumed that this choice of career was due to unprocessed experiences of mental ill health. It was thought that these unprocessed experiences might be harmful to their functioning on the job. Those times have changed. At present, these experiences are seen as a potential benefit, provided they start from the perspective of client self-management. The positive deployment of these experiences, or lived-experience expertise, in other words, has become a part of the mental healthcare professional's toolkit.

Throughout these changes in mental healthcare, Basaglia's observation, that we should not allow ourselves to be blinded by turns that seem to promise a more humane effect (Foot), still holds. They may only be apparent. The real change lies in the relationship between healthcare professional and patient; it must be one of equality and reciprocity. Lived-experience experts in teams can play a very important role in the mental healthcare professional's recovery. In the first place, it means respect for the empowered patient/citizen, and, through this, a defence of the less articulate patient/citizen's rights. It also means giving family and other citizens a say.

The key is to establish connections with and between people, despite but mainly thanks to, their differences. If we truly look at ourselves we will see that our sense of wonder at our own thinking, behaviour, fears and joys is essentially no different to others' wonder at their own thinking, behaviour, fears and joys. It is all based on getting to know each other by communicating on the basis of equality. The essentials of that communication are authenticity and openness.

We live in a time when there are more channels of communication and greater access to those channels. Used properly, social media can be an effective means of communication. I make very extensive use of social media. Among my Facebook friends, besides the patients currently on my ward, there are former patients, patients from other institutions, peer supporters, patient relatives, healthcare professionals and politicians, mostly local. This enables me to do things such as announce the projects we set up in the community. It may also lead to a chat with a critical local resident I have not yet met. I love talking to people who seem to have their reservations about what we do in the area of social integration, or are negative. I try to get them more involved in what we do, by inviting them in. In a conversation like this, you cannot change a person's negative view of people with mental ill health, but when you treat them with respect they are always reciprocally respectful, and that is a good basis for further contact.

My own recovery involved gradually getting rid of some of the ballast I had taken aboard in my studies. But I have held onto much of what I learned, and it has become an integral part of this new search for connections. I see the people in my care, their families, the local residents, my colleagues, as companions in this work. I make no distinction between them. They are all important. For that reason, I use a language that everyone understands. I stay well away from the healthcare jargon. I have no need for separate briefings, or meetings of team members only. The only reason to talk about patients in their absence is to let off steam, to feel the comfort of another's understanding when you are having problems or clashes with a patient. I see these conversations as a way to find the strength and inspiration I need to mend the broken-down communication with the patient. Here too, alternatives such as 'open dialogue', in which two healthcare professionals consult at the end of the meeting in the presence of the other participants, can point the way.

The 'us and them' feeling between community and patient disappears. We collaborate on actions in community projects on integration.

I often spread the word about quartermaking with help from patients on the ward. I see them as colleagues and companions in this, and it can lead to some very pleasing effects.

The publication of this book is something which I have worked towards with the patients and colleagues on my ward. I have spoken to them about it regularly, in group and individual talks. I have asked them if they minded my writing about the work we did together in this book. They felt honoured. Some saw it as a privilege to be in the book, because they felt heard. They were glad they could testify. Others hoped that their collaboration on the book would bring more equality for patients in the healthcare setting. I too hope that the book is of help in that way.

Like the people depicted in this book, and people with whom I collaborate (colleagues, patients and local residents), I hope that this book represents a step towards more participation, more equality, more acceptance and more inclusion. Where the next step in the process will lead, is as yet unknown. Not a grim unknown, but one that we can greet with hope...

INDEX

Farkas, M. 83, 89, 100
Feuerzeig, J. 152, 179
Flanders 20, 106, 113, 134, 165, 178;
  Enchanté 159; home care service 19
Flemish Association for Mental Health
  (now part of vzw Psyche) 112, 178
Flemish Working Group on
  Quartermaking 97, 177, 178
Foot, J. 58, 59, 60, 77, 100, 102, 103,
  180, 184
Fort, D.C. 101
Foucault, M. 4, 6, 57, 58, 100
Foudraine, J. 59
France 29, 59; see also Dicy
Franzen, J. 81, 100, 135, 180
friction 131
Froyen, B. 66, 100

gender 126
Germany 149
Gestaltungsdrang 151
Ghent 29, 89, 135, 178, 179; and
  alternative currency 161
Giezenberg, M. 101
Gigli, L. 104
Giphart, M. 6
Goffman, E. 115, 180
Gorizia 102, 103
van de Graaf, W. 180
Greyston Bakery 164, 165, 180

halfway house 121
hallucination 45, 55
happiness economics 162
Hartmann, E. 44, 45
hearing voices 37, 69, 125, 148, 171, 175;
  and drugs 32
HEE 53
Heerkens, Y. 101
Held, J.M. 68, 100, 173, 180
HIC 90
historicization 36
Hitchcock, A. 168
Höch, H. 150, 180
home support 19, 26–27, 96, 143, 172, 175
homeless 21, 22, 24–26, 92, 176–177,
  180; and childhood trauma 93; and
  mental ill health 4, 18; and psychiatric
  institution 98–99
homes of childhood see space
hope 93, 97; and connection 26, 94, 170;
  and homeless 24, 99; and long-stay

patients 62; place of 3, 10, 122, 132,
  135; provider of 4, 19, 76, 79, 88,
  124, 181
Hôpital Général 57
Hopkins, L. 77, 100
hospitable places 3, 103, 129; see also
  place
hospitality 121, 129, 131, 159–160; see
  also space
housing first 87, 97–99
Hovius, R. 60, 82, 101
Huber, M.A.S. 53, 101
Hurst, A. 159, 163, 180

identity 51, 110, 156, 180; patient 82, 83,
  111, 153–154; and stigma 49
inexpressible suffering 68, 173; see also
  Lyotard, J-F
institutional psychotherapy 59–60
integration 124, 125, 131, 133; and
  community project 185; and
  psychiatric care 19, 56
interventive care 24, 166, 171
involuntarily admission see involuntarily
  detained
involuntarily detained 23, 32, 34, 75, 89,
  145; and administrator 22; and care
  avoiders 166, 168
IPS 146, 166
Irigaray, L. 126, 132, 180
Isle of Wight 155
Italy 6, 59, 105; see also Basaglia, F.

Janssen, M. 180
Japan 4, 35
Jervis, G. 103
Johnston, D. 152–153, 179

Kal, D. 21, 24, 25, 45, 57, 60, 101, 116,
  120, 124–128, 130–136, 156, 158, 165,
  174, 178, 179, 180
Kars, M. 74, 101
Knottnerus, J.A. 101
Koning Boudewijnstichting 24, 45
KOPP see child of patient

La Fabuloserie 157
Laing, R.D. 60, 73, 101
Lausanne 152
Lauwaert, D. 43, 46
Layard, R. 162, 180
Le Carillon 159

Printed in the United States
by Baker & Taylor Publisher Services